WHAT DR. SARNO TELLS HIS TMS PATIENTS

DO:

- Resume physical activity. It won't hurt you.
- Talk to your brain: Tell it you won't take it anymore.
- Stop all physical treatments for your back—they may be blocking your recovery.

DON'T:

- Repress your anger or emotions—they can give you a pain in the back.
- Think of yourself as being injured. Psychological conditioning contributes to ongoing back pain.
- Be intimidated by back pain. You have the power to overcome it.

HEALING BACK PAIN

Using the actual case histories of his own patients, Dr. John Sarno shows why tension and unexpressed emotions—particularly anger—cause chronic back pain, and how awareness and understanding are the first steps to doing something about it.

ALSO BY JOHN E. SARNO, MD

Mind Over Back Pain
The Mindbody Prescription

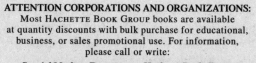

HEALING BACK PAIN

The Mind-Body Connection

JOHN E. SARNO, MD

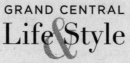

GRAND CENTRAL
Life & Style

NEW YORK · BOSTON

Copyright © 1991 by John E. Sarno, M.D.
Preface copyright © 2016 by John E. Sarno

Book design by Book design by Giorgetta Bell McRee
Cover copyright © 2017 by Hachette Book Group, Inc.

Grand Central Life & Style
Hachette Book Group
1290 Avenue of the Americas, New York, NY 10104
grandcentrallifeandstyle.com
twitter.com/grandcentralpub

Originally published in trade paperback February 1991
First oversized mass market edition: February 2018

Grand Central Life & Style is an imprint of Grand Central Publishing. The Grand Central Life & Style name and logo are trademarks of Hachette Book Group, IncGrand Central Publishing is a division of Hachette Book Group, Inc. The Grand Central Publishing name and logo is a trademark of Hachette Book Group, Inc.

The publisher is not responsible for websites (or their content) that are not owned by the publisher.

Excerpts from "Pity me not because the light of day" by Edna St. Vincent Millay. From *Collected Sonnets*, Revised and Expanded Edition, Harper & Row, 1988. Copyright © 1923, 1951 by Edna St. Vincent Millay and Norma Millay Ellis. Reprinted by permission of Elizabeth Barnett, Literary Executor.

ISBNs: 978-1-5387-1261-0 (oversize mass market); 978-0-4465-5768-9 (mass maket); 978-0-7595-2084-4 (ebook)

Printed in the United States of America

OPM

10 9 8 7 6 5

CONTENTS

PREFACE

To the 2016 Edition

I am delighted that my publisher is reissuing *Healing Back Pain*, as it affords me the opportunity to provide new readers with the historic and clinical context in which this book was first published in 1991.

As early as 1965, because of my medical specialty in physical medicine and rehabilitation, and as Director of Outpatient Services at the Rusk Institute of Rehabilitation Medicine, I cared for a greater-than-average number of patients with pain disorders, the majority with back pain. Treating back pain was frustrating and depressing for me, as I could never predict the outcome. As a physician keen on accurate diagnosis and treatment, over the years I became increasingly troubled with the fact that frequently the pattern of a patient's pain and the findings on physical examination didn't match the presumed pathology. The pain, for example, might be attributed to radiographic findings of degenerative arthritis of the joints of the last lumbar vertebra (spinal bone), but the patient often had pain in places that had nothing to do with these joints. My classical medical training taught me to consider back pain as due primarily to structural abnormalities of the spine—most commonly arthritic or disc disorders—or the result of poor posture, compression of nerves, or lack of exercise. I simply treated patients in accordance with traditional medical training.

In the early 1970s, I began to notice that the outcomes of patients with the same physical findings seemed more dependent on the degree of their faith in me as their physician rather than the physical treatment I was administering. I began to think that back pain was psychosomatic— particularly as most of the patients I saw had a history of other psychosomatic manifestations. I developed a new theory about the etiology of the pain disorder and named it TMS for Tension Myositis Syndrome, which I have since more accurately labeled the Tension Myoneural Syndrome, attributing greater prominence to the prevalence of neural symptoms rather than the involvement of inflamed muscles.

The theory, that such a very physical condition as back pain could be psychosomatic, flew in the face of convention and my medical training. Yet my own medical history and personality, my observation of thousands of patients in pain, as well as my experience during nine years as a family physician, made me receptive to the idea. I tested the theory by changing my treatment protocols and emphasizing the role of emotions in the cause of pain, and there were obvious improvements in my patients. I could begin to predict which of them would do well, and which would not. This was an exciting development in how I treated— and ultimately was able to help—my patients.

In the twenty-five years since *Healing Back Pain* was first published, the incidence and impact of back pain has increased exponentially.[1] The statistics and data are astounding. Over one hundred million people are now affected at a total cost in the United States exceeding one hundred billion dollars per year, of which two-thirds is lost to wages and reduced productivity.[2] The 2010 Global Burden of Disease study of 291 conditions ranked low back pain as the highest cause of disability and sixth in terms of overall burden.[3] When measured in terms of years lived with disability (DALYS = Disability Adjusted Life Years), the incidence of low back pain increased an estimated 43% between 1990 and 2010, leading to the prediction that living with disability will soon outnumber years of life lost to early death.[4]

As the incidence of back pain increased, the pharmacology industry introduced new opioid pain medications and quadrupled its sales of synthetic opiates. This may have been partly driven by the industry, but many patients have welcomed and encouraged it, perhaps in response to the belief that modern medicine has the power to cure all illnesses[5] or out of the wish to alleviate the desperation that results from the reality of living with chronic pain and disability. Put simply, the chronic pain epidemic impacts the lives of individuals and families by adding innumerable physical and emotional challenges to the possibility of leading satisfied, comfortable, and contented lives.

Another major shift since 1991 is that individuals increasingly engage in their own health care decisions—and there has been a fundamental change in our understanding of wellness. The public now has unprecedented access to health information, especially through the internet, and patients have become their own health advocates. There has also been a notable increase in the public's health literacy, reflected in the level of sophistication of widely circulated publications and the establishment of centers and programs devoted to health and wellness in communities of all sizes.

A shift in authority from the physician to patient, in large part because of access to clinical information on the web,[6] has resulted in individuals now being thought of as consumers who should take charge of their health.[7] The fact that TMS is a diagnosis for which the treatment is education fits right into this more modern way of thinking. It is my contention that the chronic pain epidemic could be reversed if more physicians and patients understood TMS.

In 1992, the scientific community acknowledged the role of emotions on physical health when Congress mandated the National Institutes of Health to open an Office of Complementary and Alternative Medicine, which moved mind-body research and practice closer to the medical mainstream. This mandate has stimulated government-sponsored and privately funded research, as well as added mind-body medicine to medical school curricula.[8] However, psychosomatic medicine is still not being adequately taught to physicians other than psychiatrists and, ironically, it is physicians such as internists, orthopedists, rheumatologists, gastroenterologists, dermatologists, etc. who must make the psychosomatic diagnosis before it can be adequately treated by a psychiatrist or psychologist. Furthermore, the modern health care system, based as it is on a rigorous corporate model, does not allow for adequate time to be spent with patients to elicit the basis for the symptoms and poses another impediment to stemming the tide of chronic pain.

During my professional life, particularly over the last fifty years, the medical culture that rewards specialization, efficiency, and hard data has forced the contemporary physician to distance himself from the patient. The clinical examination and the emotional status of the patient are often compromised and it is difficult for the contemporary physician to engage the patient in a conversation about life, hopes, disappointments, and ambitions.

As this trend in contemporary medical culture has taken hold, physicians are still not trained to recognize psychosomatic disorders. They are trained to explain all physical disorders with physical structural reasons and, therefore, not to consider the role of emotions in the etiology of physical disorders. As a consequence, patients with back pain do not receive appropriate treatment, which would mandate paying attention to emotional phenomena. According to contemporary diagnostics, physical disorders are purely the consequence of structural, physical maladies. Psychosomatic etiology, therefore, has no role in the diagnosis of pain disorders, and the physician's training continues to associate medical practice with matters of the body exclusively. The patient is viewed as a machine controlled by several systems, omitting the person's psychology entirely as one of those systems. This omission in the physician's portfolio has been a leading factor in the epidemiological increase of pain disorders.

When I wrote *Healing Back Pain*, my intention was to describe a very common, almost universal, pain disorder to professionals and the public. I never anticipated that merely reading the book would relieve so many patients of their pain. Yet I continue to receive communications from all over the world reporting that reading the book was sufficient to heal the pain and gain psychological insights. These insights may also protect patients from other psychophysiological disorders.

I have been astounded and impressed at the healing

power of knowledge, which became a guiding principle and practice in my treatment program with TMS patients. I am, of course, forever grateful for their open accounts of their physical and psychological struggles as well as their willingness to put their faith in me by accepting and confirming a theory that for many seemed preposterous. Without my patients and the many who have come forward to share their struggles and successes with chronic pain, I would not have had the opportunity to develop an even more robust TMS theory, which continues to help large numbers of people with chronic, debilitating pain.

Psychosomatic disorders are an inescapable manifestation of the human experience. Almost everyone has had some psychosomatic symptoms. I view the reissue of *Healing Back Pain* as an essential event illustrating that empowered pain sufferers demand treatment for their pain that considers the whole person as a complex emotional and physical being. My hope is that my colleagues will continue to study and contribute to our understanding of the diagnosis and treatment of psychophysiological disorders.

John E. Sarno, M.D.
New York City
August 2016

NOTES

1. J.K. Freburger, G.M. Holmes, R.P. Agans, A.M. Jackman, J.D. Darter, A.S. Wallace, L.D. Castel, W.D. Kalsbeek, and T.S. Carey, "The Rising Prevalence of Chronic Low Back Pain," *Archives of Internal Medicine* 169, no. 3 (Feb. 2009): 251–258.

2. J.N. Katz, "Lumbar Disc Disorders and Low Back Pain: Socio-Economic Factors and Consequences," *The Journal of Bone and Joint*

Surgery Am. 88, no. 2 (Apr. 2006): 21-24; S. Dagenais, J. Caro, and S. Haldeman, "A Systematic Review of Low Back Pain Cost of Illness Studies in the United States and Internationally," *The Spine Journal* 8, no. 1 (Jan–Feb. 2008): 8–20; W.T. Crow and D.R. Willis, "Estimating Cost of Care for Patients with Acute Low Back Pain: A Retrospective Review of Patient Records," *The Journal of the American Osteopathic Association* 109, no. 4 (Apr. 2009): 229–233.

3. Damian Hoy, et al, "The Global Burden of Low Back Pain: Estimates from the Global Burden of Disease 2010 Study," *Annals of the Rheumatic Diseases* 73, no. 6 (2014): 968–974.

4. J.N. Smith, *Epic Measures: One Doctor. Seven Billion Patients* (New York: HarperCollins Publishers, 2015).

5. Celine Gounder, M.D., "Who is Responsible for the Pain-Pill Epidemic?" *The New Yorker* (Nov. 8, 2013).

6. P. Hartzband and J. Groopman, "How Medical Care is Being Corrupted," *The New York Times* (Nov. 18, 2014).

7. Eric Topol, M.D., *The Patient Will See You Now: The Future of Medicine is in Your Hands* (New York: Basic Books, 2015).

8. J.H. Young, "The Development of the Office of Alternative Medicine in the National Institutes of Health 1991–1996," *Bulletin of the History of Medicine* 72, no. 2 (Summer 1998): 279–298; V. Brower, "Mind-Body Research Moves Towards the Mainstream," *EMBO Reports* 7, no. 4 (Apr. 2006): 358–361.

INTRODUCTION

This book is the successor to *Mind Over Back Pain,* which was published in 1984. It described a medical disorder known as the Tension Myositis Syndrome (TMS), which I have had reason to believe is the major cause of the common syndromes of pain involving the neck, shoulders, back, buttocks, and limbs. In the years since that first publication, I have further developed and clarified my concepts about how to diagnose and treat TMS, hence the necessity for this book.

Over the years, the increasing incidence of these pain syndromes has created a public health problem of impressive proportions. One continues to see the statistic that somewhere around 80 percent of the population have a history of one of these painful conditions. An article in *Forbes* magazine in August 1986 reported that $56 billion are spent annually to deal with the consequences of this ubiquitous medical disorder. It is the first cause of worker absenteeism in this country and ranks second behind respiratory infections as a reason for a doctor visit.

All this has happened in the past thirty years. Why? After a few million years of evolution, has the American back suddenly become incompetent? Why are so many people prone to back injury? And why has the medical profession proven so helpless to stem the epidemic?

It is this book's purpose to answer those and many other questions about this widespread problem. The thesis will be advanced that, like all epidemics, this one is the result of medicine's failure to recognize the nature of the disease—that is, to make an accurate diagnosis. The plague ravaged the world because no one knew anything about bacteriology or epidemiology at the time. It may be hard to believe that highly sophisticated twentieth-century medicine cannot properly identify the cause of something so simple and common as these pain disorders, but physicians and medical researchers are, after all, still human and, therefore, not all-knowing and, most important, subject to the enduring weakness of bias.

The pertinent bias here is that these common pain syndromes must be the result of structural abnormalities of the spine or chemically or mechanically induced deficiencies of muscle. Of equal importance is another bias held by conventional medicine that emotions do not induce physiologic change. Experience with TMS contradicts both biases. The disorder is a benign (though painful) physiologic aberration of soft tissue (not the spine), and it is caused by an emotional process.

I first appreciated the magnitude of this problem in 1965 when I joined the staff of what is now known as the Howard A. Rusk Institute of Rehabilitation Medicine at New York University Medical Center as director of outpatient services. It was my first introduction to large numbers of patients with neck, shoulder, back, and buttock pain. Conventional medical training had taught me that these pains were primarily due to a variety of structural abnormalities of the spine, most commonly arthritic and disc disorders, or to a vague group of muscle conditions attributed to poor posture, underexercise, overexertion, and the like. Pain in the legs or arms was presumed due to compression (pinching) of nerves. However, it was not at all clear how these abnormalities actually produced the pain.

The rationale for the treatment prescribed was equally perplexing. Treatment included injections, deep heat in the form of ultrasound, massage, and exercise. No one was sure what these regimens were supposed to do, but they seemed to help in some cases. It was said that the exercise strengthened the abdominal and back muscles and that this somehow supported the spine and prevented pain.

The experience of treating these patients was frustrating and depressing; one could never predict the outcome. Further, it was troubling to realize that the pattern of pain and physical examination findings often did not correlate with the presumed reason for the pain. For example, pain might be attributed to degenerative arthritic changes at the lower end of the spine, but the patient might have pain in places that had nothing to do with the bones in that area. Or someone might have a lumbar disc that was herniated to the left and have pain in the right leg.

Along with doubt about the accuracy of conventional diagnoses, there came the realization that the primary tissue involved was muscle, specifically the muscles of the neck, shoulders, back, and buttocks. But even more important was the observation that 88 percent of the people seen had histories of such things as tension or migraine headache, heartburn, hiatus hernia, stomach ulcer, colitis, spastic colon, irritable bowel syndrome, hay fever, asthma, eczema, and a variety of other disorders, all of which were strongly suspected of being related to tension. It seemed logical to conclude that their painful muscle condition might also be induced by tension. Hence, the Tension Myositis Syndrome (TMS). (*Myo* means "muscle"; *Tension Myositis Syndrome* is defined here as a change of state in the muscle that is painful.)

When that theory was put to the test and patients were treated accordingly, there was an improvement in treatment results. In fact, it was then possible to predict with some accuracy which patients would do well and which would probably fail. That was the beginning of the diagnostic and therapeutic program described in this book.

It should be emphasized that this book does not describe a "new approach" to the treatment of back pain. TMS is a *new diagnosis* and therefore must be treated in a manner appropriate to the diagnosis. When medicine learned that bacteria were the cause of many infections, it looked for ways to deal with germs—hence the antibiotics. If emotional factors are responsible for someone's back pain, one must look for a proper therapeutic technique. Clearly, there is no logic to traditional physical treatment. Instead, experience has shown that the only successful and permanent way to treat the problem is by teaching patients to understand what they have. To the uninitiated, that may not make much sense but it should become clear as one reads on.

Is this holistic medicine? Unfortunately, what has come to be known as holistic medicine is a jumble of science, pseudoscience, and folklore. Anything that is outside mainstream medicine may be accepted as holistic, but more accurately described, the predominant idea is that one must treat the "whole person," a wise concept that is generally neglected by contemporary medicine. But that should not give license to identify anything as holistic that defies medical convention.

Perhaps *holistic* should be defined as that which includes consideration of both the emotional and structural aspects of health and illness. In accepting this definition, one does not reject the scientific method. On the contrary, it becomes increasingly important to require proof and replication of results when one adds the very difficult emotional dimension to the medical equation.

Therefore, this is not holistic medicine as it is popularly conceived. I hope it is an example of good medicine—accurate diagnosis and effective treatment, and good science—conclusions based on observation, verified by experience. Though the cause of TMS is tension, the diagnosis is made on physical and not psychological grounds, in the tradition of clinical medicine.

All physicians should be practitioners of "holistic medicine" in the sense that they recognize the interaction between mind and body. To leave the emotional dimension out of the study of health and illness is poor medicine and poor science.

There is an important point to be emphasized: Though TMS is induced by emotional phenomena, it is a physical disorder. It must be diagnosed by a physician, someone who is capable of recognizing both the physical and psychological dimensions of the condition. Psychologists may suspect that patients' symptoms are emotionally induced but, not trained in physical diagnosis, cannot say with certainty that they have TMS. Since very few physicians are trained to recognize a disorder whose roots are psychological, TMS falls between the cracks, as it were, and patients go undiagnosed. It is particularly important that the diagnosis be made by a physician to avoid the pejorative conclusion that the pain is "all in the head."

What do doctors think of this diagnosis? It is unlikely that most physicians are aware of it. I have written a number of medical papers and chapters for textbooks on the subject, but they have reached a limited medical audience, primarily physicians working in the field of physical medicine and rehabilitation. In recent years it has become impossible to have medical papers on TMS accepted for publication, undoubtedly because these concepts fly in the face of contemporary medical dogma. For those physicians who might see this book, I would point out that it is more complete than any of the papers I have published and will be useful to them despite the fact that it is written for a general audience.

Judging by the reactions of doctors in my immediate environment, most physicians will either ignore or reject the diagnosis. A few doctors in my own specialty say that they see the validity of the diagnosis but find it difficult to treat such patients. One hopes that the younger generation of physicians will be more capable of dealing with this kind of problem. It is one of the intentions of this book to reach those young doctors.

What of those readers who are having neck, shoulder, back, or buttock pain and think they may have TMS? A book cannot substitute for a doctor, and it is not my intention to diagnose and treat through this book. I consider it unethical and immoral to hold oneself out as a physician through a book or a DVD. Pain syndromes must always be properly studied to rule out serious disorders such as cancer, tumors, bone disease, and many other conditions. If one has persistent pain anywhere, it is imperative to see a doctor so that appropriate examinations and tests can be done.

The primary purpose of this book is to raise consciousness both inside and outside the field of medicine, because these common pain syndromes represent a major public health problem that will not be solved until there is a change in the medical perception of their cause.

Having stated the purpose of the book, I would be less than candid if I did not report that many readers of its predecessor, *Mind Over Back Pain,* reported amelioration or complete resolution of symptoms. This substantiates the idea that it is identification with and knowledge of the disorder that are the critical therapeutic factors.

Science requires that all new ideas be validated by experience and replication. Before new concepts can be generally accepted, they must be proven beyond all doubt. It is essential that the ideas advanced in this book be subjected to research study. In the tradition of scientific medicine, I invite my colleagues to verify or correct my work. What they ought not do is ignore it, for the problem of back pain is too great and the need for a solution imperative.

HEALING
BACK PAIN

1

The Manifestations of TMS

I have never seen a patient with pain in the neck, shoulders, back, or buttocks who didn't believe that the pain was due to an injury, a "hurt" brought on by some physical activity. "I hurt myself while running (playing basketball, tennis, bowling)." "The pain started after I lifted my little girl" or "when I tried to open a stuck window." "Ten years ago I was involved in a hit-from-behind auto accident, and I have had recurrent back pain ever since."

The idea that pain means injury or damage is deeply ingrained in the American consciousness. Of course, if the pain starts while one is engaged in a physical activity, it's difficult not to attribute the pain to the activity. (As we shall see later, that is often deceiving.) But this pervasive concept of the vulnerability of the back, of ease of injury, is nothing less than a medical catastrophe for the American public, which now has an army of semidisabled men and women whose lives are significantly restricted by the fear of doing further damage or bringing on the dreaded pain again. One often hears,

"I'm afraid of hurting myself again, so I'm going to be very careful of what I do."

In good faith, this idea has been fostered by the medical profession and other healers for years. It has been assumed that neck, shoulder, back, and buttock pain is due to injury or disease of the spine and associated structures or incompetence of muscles and ligaments surrounding these structures—without scientific validation of these diagnostic concepts.

On the other hand, I have had gratifying success in the treatment of these disorders for seventeen years based on a very different diagnosis. It has been my observation that the majority of these pain syndromes are the result of a condition in the muscles, nerves, tendons, and ligaments brought on by tension. And the point has been proven by the very high rate of success achieved with a treatment program that is simple, rapid, and thorough.

Medicine's preoccupation with the spine draws on fundamental medical philosophy and training. Modern medicine has been primarily mechanical and structural in orientation. The body is viewed as an exceedingly complex machine and illness as a malfunction in the machine brought about by infection, trauma, inherited defects, degeneration, and, of course, cancer. At the same time, medical science has had a love affair with the laboratory, believing that nothing is valid unless it can be demonstrated in that arena. No one would dispute the essential role the laboratory has played in medical progress (witness penicillin and insulin, for example). Unfortunately, some things are difficult to study in the laboratory. One of these is the mind and its organ, the brain. The emotions do not lend themselves to test-tube experiments and measurement, and so modern medical science has chosen to ignore them, but-tressed by the conviction that emotions have little to do with health and illness anyway. Hence, the majority of practicing physicians do not consider that emotions play a significant role in *causing* physical disorders, though many would ac-knowledge that they might aggravate a "physically" caused illness. In general, physicians feel uncomfortable in deal-ing with a problem that is related to the emotions. They tend to make a sharp division between "the things of the mind" and "the things of the body," and only feel comfort-able with the latter.

Peptic ulcer of the duodenum is a good example. Al-though some physicians would dispute the idea, there is fairly wide acceptance among practicing doctors that ul-cers are caused primarily by "tension." Contrary to logic, however, the major focus in treatment is "medical," not "psychological," and drugs are prescribed to neutralize or prevent the secretion of acid. But failure to treat the pri-mary cause of the disorder is poor medicine; it is symp-tomatic treatment, something we were warned about in medical school. But since most physicians see their role only as treating the body, the psychological part of the problem is neglected, even though it's the basic cause. In fairness, some physicians make an attempt to say some-thing about tension, but it's often of a superficial nature, like, "You ought to take it easy; you're working too hard."

Pain syndromes look so "physical" it is particularly difficult for doctors to consider the possibility that they might be caused by psychological factors, and so they cling to the structural explanation. In doing so, however, they are chiefly responsible for the pain epidemic that now exists in this country.

If structural abnormalities don't cause pain in the neck, shoulder, back, and buttocks, what does? Studies and clinical experience of many years suggest that these common pain syndromes are the result of a physiologic alteration in certain muscles, nerves, tendons, and ligaments that is called the Tension Myositis Syndrome (TMS). It is a harmless but potentially very painful disorder that is the result of specific, common emotional situations. It is the purpose of this book to describe TMS in detail.

The ensuing sections of this chapter will discuss who gets it, in what parts of the body it occurs, the various patterns of pain, and the overall impact of TMS on people's health and daily lives. Following chapters will talk about the psychology of TMS (which is where it all begins), its physiology, and how it is treated. Conventional diagnosis and treatment will be reviewed, and I will conclude with a chapter on the important interaction between mind and body in matters of health and illness.

WHO GETS TMS?

One might almost say that TMS is a cradle-to-grave disorder, since it does occur in children, though probably not until the age of five or six. Its manifestation in children is, of course, different from what occurs in adults. I am convinced that what are referred to as "growing pains" in children are manifestations of TMS.

The cause of "growing pains" has never been identified, but physicians have always been comfortable in reassuring mothers that the condition is harmless. It occurred to me one day while listening to a young mother describe her daughter's severe leg pain in the middle of the night that what the child had experienced was very much like an adult attack of sciatica, and since this was clearly one of the most common manifestations of TMS, "growing pains" might very well represent TMS in children.

Little wonder that no one has been able to explain the nature of "growing pains," since TMS is a condition that usually leaves no physical evidence of its presence. There is a temporary constriction of blood vessels, bringing on the symptoms, and then all returns to normal.

The emotional stimulus for the attack in children is no different from that in adults—anxiety. One might say that the attack in a child is a paranightmare. It is a substitute for a nightmare, a command decision by the mind to produce a physical reaction rather than have the individual experience a painful emotion, which is what happens in adults as well.

At the other end of the spectrum, I have seen the syndrome in men and women in their eighties. There appears to be no age limit, and why would there be? As long as one can generate emotions, one is susceptible to the disorder.

What are the ages when it is most common, and can we learn anything from those statistics? In a follow-up survey carried out in 1982, 177 patients were interviewed as to their then current status following treatment for TMS. (See page 103 for results of the survey.) We learned that 77 percent of the patients fell between the ages of thirty and sixty, 9 percent were in their twenties, and there were only four teenagers (2 percent). At the other end of the spectrum, only 7 percent were in their sixties and 4 percent in their seventies.

These statistics suggest very strongly that the cause of most back pain is emotional, for the years between thirty and sixty are the ages that fall into what I would call the years of responsibility. This is the period in one's life when one is under the most strain to succeed, to provide and excel, and it is logical that this is when one would experience the highest incidence of TMS. Further, if degenerative changes in the spine (osteoarthritis, disc degeneration and herniation, facet arthrosis, and spinal stenosis, for instance) were a primary cause of back pain, these statistics wouldn't fit at all. In that case, a gradual increase in incidence from the twenties on would occur, with the highest incidence in the oldest people. To be sure, this is only circumstantial evidence, but it is highly suggestive.

So the answer to the question "Who gets TMS?" is "Anybody." But it is certainly most common in the middle years of life, the years of responsibility. Let's now take a look at how TMS manifests itself.

WHERE DOES TMS MANIFEST ITSELF?

Muscle

The primary tissue involved in TMS is muscle, hence the original name *myositis* (as mentioned, *myo* stands for "muscle"). The only muscles in the body that are susceptible to TMS are those in the back of the neck, the entire back, and the buttocks, known collectively as *postural muscles*. They are so named because they maintain the correct posture of the head and trunk and contribute to the effective use of the arms.

Postural muscles have a higher proportion of "slow twitch" muscle fibers than limb muscles, making them more efficient for endurance activity, which is what is required of them. Whether or not this is the reason why TMS is restricted to this group of muscles we do not know. It is possible, though, since the muscles most frequently involved have the most important jobs. These are the buttock muscles, known anatomically as *gluteal muscles*. Their job is to keep the trunk upright on the legs, to prevent it from falling forward or to either side. Statistically, the low back–buttock area is the most common location for TMS.

Just above the buttocks are the lumbar muscles (in the small of the back), often involved simultaneously with buttock muscles. Occasionally the gluteal or lumbar muscles are affected separately. Roughly two-thirds of TMS patients will have their major pain in this area.

Second in order of frequency of involvement are the neck and shoulder muscles. The pain is usually in the side of the neck and the top of the shoulder, in the upper trapezius muscle.

TMS can occur anywhere else in the back, between the shoulders and low back, but does so far less frequently than in the two areas mentioned.

Generally a patient will complain of pain in one of these prime areas, as, for example, in the left buttock or the right shoulder, but the physical examination will reveal something else of great interest and importance. In virtually every patient with TMS, one finds tenderness when pressure is applied (palpation) to muscles in three parts of the back: the outer aspect of both buttocks (and sometimes to the entire buttock), the muscles in the lumbar area, and both upper trapezius (shoulder) muscles. This consistent pattern is important, because it supports the hypothesis that the pain syndrome originates in the brain rather than in some structural abnormality of the spine or incompetence of the muscle.

Nerve

The second type of tissue to be implicated in this syndrome is nerve, specifically what are known as *peripheral nerves*. Those most frequently affected are located, as might be expected, in close proximity to the muscles that are involved most often.

The sciatic nerve is located deep in the buttock muscle (one on each side); lumbar spinal nerves are under the lumbar paraspinal muscles; the cervical spinal nerves and brachial plexus are under the upper trapezius (shoulder) muscles. These are the nerves most frequently affected in TMS.

In fact, TMS looks like a *regional* process, rather than one aimed at specific structures. So when it affects a given area, all the tissues suffer oxygen deprivation so that one may experience both muscle and nerve pain.

Varying kinds of pain may result when muscle and/or nerve are affected. It may be sharp, aching, burning, shocklike, or it may feel like pressure. In addition to pain, nerve involvement may produce feelings of pins and needles, tingling and/or numbness, and sometimes sensations of weakness in the legs or arms. In some cases there is measurable muscle weakness. The latter can be documented with electromyographic studies (EMG). EMG abnormalities are often cited as evidence of nerve damage due to structural compression, but in fact, EMG changes are very common in TMS and usually reveal involvement of many more nerves than could be explained by a structural abnormality.

Lumbar spinal and sciatic nerve symptoms are in the legs, for that is where those nerves are going. Involvement of cervical spinal nerves and brachial plexus causes symptoms in the arms and hands. Traditional diagnoses attribute leg pain to a herniated disc and arm pain to a "pinched nerve." (See chapter 5.)

TMS may involve any of the nerves in the neck, shoulders, back, and buttocks, sometimes producing unusual pain patterns. One of the most frightening is chest pain. One immediately thinks of the heart when there is chest pain, and, indeed, it is always important to be sure that there is nothing wrong with that organ. Once having done so, one should keep in mind that spinal nerves in the upper back may be suffering mild oxygen deprivation because of TMS and that this may be the source of the pain. These nerves serve the front of the trunk as well as the back, hence the chest pain.

Remember: Always consult a regular physician in order to rule out serious disorders. This book is not intended as a guide to self-diagnosis. Its purpose is to describe a clinical entity, TMS.

One may suspect the presence of nerve involvement in TMS through the patient's history, the physical examination, or both. Sciatic pain may affect any part of the leg except the upper, front thigh. There is considerable variability depending on how much of the nerve trunk is affected by oxygen debt. As noted above, the person may also complain of other strange feelings and of weakness.

On physical examination, the tendon reflexes and muscle strength are tested to determine whether oxygen deprivation has irritated the nerve sufficiently to interfere with the transmission of motor impulses. Similarly, sensory tests are done (for example, ability to feel a pinprick) to determine the integrity of the sensory fibers in the involved nerve. The major virtue of documenting sensory or motor deficits is to be able to discuss them with patients and reassure them that feelings of weakness, numbness, or tingling are quite harmless.

The so-called straight leg–raising test is always done when a patient is examined, though for different reasons, depending on the examiner. If there is a great deal of soreness in the buttocks, the patient will be unable to elevate the straightened leg very far and then only with a great deal of pain. The pain may be due to the muscle, the sciatic nerve, or both. What the sign does not mean in the majority of cases is that there is a herniated disc "pressing on the sciatic nerve," as patients are often told.

When there is a shoulder-arm pain syndrome, one does similar tests on the arm and hand.

Sometimes patients have pain on two sides; this is of no particular significance. People will also often report that in addition to having the major pain in the right buttock and leg, for example, they have some intermittent pain in the neck or one of the shoulders. This is not unexpected, since TMS may involve any or all of the postural muscles.

Tendons and Ligaments

Following the publication of my first book describing TMS, I gradually became aware that a variety of tendonalgias (pain in tendons or ligaments) were probably part of the syndrome of tension myositis. The term *myositis* was fast becoming obsolete, it having been determined many years before that nerves could be implicated in TMS, as just described. Now I was beginning to realize that still another type of tissue might be part of the process, and as time went by, this conclusion became more and more inescapable.

What first attracted attention were reports from treated patients: In addition to the disappearance of back pain, their tendon pain (for example, tennis elbow) often left as well. As is well known, tennis elbow is one of the most common of the disorders called *tendonitis*. Generally, it is assumed that these painful tendons are inflamed, presumably because of excessive activity. The routine treatment is anti-inflammatory medication and activity restriction.

Having been alerted to the possibility that these painful tendons might be part of TMS, I began to suggest to patients that their tendonitis might also disappear if they allowed it to occupy the same place in their thinking as the back pain. The results were encouraging, and over time, my confidence in the diagnosis increased. I am now prepared to say that tendonalgia is often an integral part of TMS and in some cases is its primary manifestation.

It has become apparent that the elbow is not the most common site of tendonalgia. In my experience, the knee has that distinction. Some of the usual diagnoses for knee

11

pain are chondromalacia, unstable knee cap, and trauma. However, the examination discloses that there is tenderness of one or more of the tendons and ligaments surrounding the knee joint, and the pain usually disappears along with the back pain.

Another common place is the foot and ankle, either the top or bottom of the foot, or the Achilles tendon. Common foot diagnoses are neuroma, bone spur, plantar fasciitis, flat feet, and trauma due to excessive physical activity.

The shoulder is another location for TMS tendonalgia; the usual structural diagnosis is bursitis or rotator cuff disorder. Again, there is usually easily identified tenderness on palpation of a tendon in the shoulder. Wrist tendons are not uncommonly involved. It is possible that what is known as carpal tunnel syndrome may also be part of TMS, but this cannot be stated without further observation and study.

Recently I saw a patient who had developed pain in a new location after a minor accident. She said the pain was in her hip and that X-rays showed that there was arthritis of the hip joints, more on the side where she was having pain, and she had been told that this was the cause of her pain. She had proven to be highly susceptible to TMS in the past, so I suggested she come in for an examination. The X-rays showed a very modest amount of arthritic change in the joint in question, about what would be expected in someone of her age. She had excellent range of motion of the joint and no pain on weight bearing or movement of the leg. When I asked her to touch the exact spot where she felt the pain, she identified a small area where the tendon of a muscle attaches to bone, well above the hip joint; it was tender to pressure. I told her I thought she had TMS tendonalgia, and the pain left in a few days.

Hip tendonalgia is most commonly attributed to what is called *trochanteric bursitis*. That diagnosis was not made on this occasion, because the location of pain was above the trochanter, the bony prominence that can be felt at the upper, outer aspect of the hip.

TMS can manifest itself in a variety of locations, and it tends to move around, particularly if something is being done to combat the disorder. Patients often report pain in a new location as the old one gets better. It is as though the brain is unwilling to give up this convenient strategy for diverting attention away from the realm of the emotions. It is, therefore, particularly important for the patient to know where all the possible locations of pain are. My patients are routinely instructed to call me when they develop new pain so that we can determine whether it is part of TMS.

In summary, TMS involves three types of tissue: muscle, nerve, and tendon-ligaments. Let us now look at how TMS manifests itself.

PATIENT CONCEPTS OF CAUSE AND TYPE OF ONSET

When first seen, most people are under the impression that they have been suffering from the long-term results of an injury, a degenerative process, a congenital abnormality, or some deficiency in the strength or flexibility of their muscles. The idea of injury is probably the most pervasive. This often ties in with the circumstances under which the pain begins.

According to a survey we did a number of years ago, 40 percent of a typical group of patients reported that the pain began in association with some kind of physical incident. For some it was a minor automobile accident, usually the hit-from-behind type. Falls, on the ice or down steps, was common. Lifting a heavy object or straining was another, and, of course, running, tennis, golf, or basketball was often blamed. The pain began anywhere from minutes to hours or days after the incident, raising some important questions about the nature of the pain. Some of the reported incidents were trivial, such as bending over to pick up a toothbrush or twisting to reach into a cupboard, but the ensuing pain might be just as excruciating as that experienced by someone who was trying to lift a refrigerator.

I recall a young man who was sitting at his office desk writing and experienced a spasm in his low back so severe and persistent that he had to be taken home by ambulance. The next forty-eight hours were agonizing; he couldn't move without setting off a new wave of spasm.

How can such excruciating pain be set off by this great variety of physical incidents? In view of the different degrees of severity of the physical incidents and the great variation in when the pain begins after the incident, the conclusion is that the physical happening was not the cause of the pain but was merely a *trigger*. Many patients apparently don't need a trigger; the pain just comes on gradually or they awaken with it in the morning. In the survey mentioned above, 60 percent fell into that category.

The idea that physical incidents are triggers is reinforced by the fact that there is no way to distinguish between those pains that start gradually and those that begin dramatically in terms of subsequent severity or longevity of the attack. All of this makes perfect sense when one considers the nature of TMS. Despite the perception of injury, patients are not injured. The physical occurrence has given the brain the opportunity to begin an attack of TMS.

There is another reason to doubt the role of injury in these attacks of back pain. One of the most powerful systems that has evolved over the millions of years of life on this planet is the biologic capacity for healing, for restoration. Our body parts tend to heal very quickly when they are injured. Even the largest bone in the body, the femur, only takes six weeks to heal. And during that process, there is pain for only a very short time. It is illogical to think that an injury that occurred two months ago might still be causing pain, not to mention one of two or ten years ago. And yet people have been so thoroughly indoctrinated with the idea of persistent injury that they accept it without question.

Invariably those patients who have a gradual onset of pain will attribute it to a physical incident that may have occurred years before, like an automobile or skiing accident. Because in their minds back pain is "physical"— that is, *structural*—it must be due to an injury. As far as they are concerned, there *has to be* a physical cause.

This idea is one of the great impediments in the way of recovery. It must be resolved in the patient's mind or the pain will persist. Gradually, patients need to begin to think psychologically; and, indeed, once the diagnosis of TMS is made, it is common for patients to begin to recall

all of the psychological things that were going on in their lives when acute attacks occurred, like starting a new job, getting married, an illness in the family, a financial crisis, and so on. Or the patient will acknowledge that he or she has always been a worrier, overly conscientious and responsible, compulsive and perfectionistic. This is the beginning of wisdom, the start of the process of putting things into proper perspective. In this case, it is the recognition that there are physical disorders that play a psychological role in human biology. Not to be aware of that fact is to doom oneself to perpetual pain and disability.

THE CHARACTER OF ONSET

The Acute Attack

Perhaps the most common, and undoubtedly the most frightening, manifestation of TMS is the acute attack. It usually comes out of the blue, and the pain is often excruciating, as described in the case of the young man above. The most common location for these attacks is the low back, involving the lumbar (small of the back) muscles, the buttock muscles, or both. Any movement brings on a new wave of terrible pain, so the condition is very upsetting, to say the least. It is clear that the involved muscles have gone into spasm. Spasm is a state of extreme contraction (tightening, tensing) of the muscles, an abnormal condition that may be horrifically painful. Most everyone has experienced a leg or foot cramp (charley horse), which is the same thing, except that the cramp will stop as soon as the involved muscle is stretched. The spasm of an attack of TMS does not let up. When it begins to ease, any movement can start it up again.

As will be described in the physiology chapter (see page 70), I believe that oxygen deprivation is responsible for the spasm as well as other kinds of pain characteristic of TMS. It is likely that common leg cramps also result from oxygen deprivation, which is why they usually occur in bed when the circulation of blood is slowed down and there is liable to be a temporary, minor state of reduced oxygenation in the leg muscles. Blood flow can be quickly restored to normal with muscle contraction. With TMS, however, reduced blood flow is continued by action of the autonomic nerves, and the abnormal muscle state persists.

People often report that at the moment of onset, they hear some kind of noise, a crack, a snap, or a pop. Patients often use the phrase "My back went out." They are sure that something has broken. In fact, nothing breaks, but the patient will swear that there has been some kind of structural damage. The noise is a mystery. It may be that it is similar to the noise elicited by a manipulation of the spine, which is a kind of "cracking the knuckles" of the joints of the spinal bones. One thing is clear—the noise indicates nothing harmful.

Though the low back is the most common location for an acute attack, it can occur anywhere in the neck, shoulders, or upper and lower back. Wherever it occurs, it is the most painful thing I know of in clinical medicine, which is ironic because it is completely harmless.

Not uncommonly, the trunk is distorted by one of these attacks. It may be bent forward or to the side, or a bit of

17

both. The precise reason for and mechanism of this is not known. Naturally, it's very disturbing but it has no special significance.

These episodes last for varying periods of time and invariably leave the person with a sense of dread and apprehension. The common perception is that something terrible has happened and that it is important to be very careful not to do anything that will injure the back and bring on another attack.

If the low back pain is accompanied by pain in the leg, or sciatica, there is even greater concern and apprehension, for this raises the possibility of the herniated disc and the possibility of surgery. In this media-dominated age, very few people have not heard of herniated discs, and the idea arouses great anxiety, resulting in greater pain. If, in the course of medical investigation, imaging studies show a herniation, the apprehension is multiplied even further. And if there should be feelings of numbness or tingling in the leg or foot and/or weakness, all of which can occur with TMS, because of burgeoning fear, the conditions for a very protracted episode of pain are defined. As will be discussed later, herniated discs are rarely the cause of the pain (see page 118).

There is not a great deal one can do to speed the resolution of such an episode. If the person is fortunate enough to know what is going on, that this is only a muscle spasm and there is nothing structurally wrong, the attack will be short-lived. But this is rarely the case. I advise my patients to remain quietly in bed, perhaps take a strong painkiller, and not agonize over what has happened. They are further instructed to keep testing their ability to move around and not assume they are going to be immobilized for days or weeks. If one can overcome one's apprehension, the duration of the attack will be considerably shorter.

The Slow Onset of Pain

In over half the cases of TMS, the pain begins gradually—there is no dramatic episode. In some cases, there is no physical incident to which one can attribute the pain. In others, onset of pain may follow a physical happening, but hours, days, or even weeks later. This pattern is fairly common after a so-called whiplash incident. A car is struck from behind and your head snaps back. Examination and X-rays do not reveal a fracture or dislocation, but sometime thereafter, pain begins, usually in the neck and shoulders, occasionally in the mid or low back. Pain in an arm or hand may also occur and, like sciatica, arouses a great deal of anxiety. Sometimes the pain begins in the neck and shoulders and then moves down to involve the rest of the back. If one knows that this is TMS, the course may be relatively brief. If some sort of structural diagnosis is made, symptoms may continue for many months, despite treatment.

THE TIMING OF ONSET

Acute attack or slow onset, why does the pain begin when it does? Remember, the physical incident, no matter how dramatic, is a trigger. The answer, of course, is to be found in one's psychological state. Sometimes the reason is obvious—a financial or health crisis, or something one ordinarily thinks of as a happy occasion, like getting married or the birth of a child. I have had a number of highly competitive people whose pain began in the course of athletic competition, like a tennis match. Naturally, they assumed that they had "hurt" themselves. When they realized they had TMS, they admitted how very anxious they had been about the competition.

It is not the occasion itself but the degree of anxiety or anger that it generates that determines if there will be a physical reaction. The important thing is the emotion generated and *repressed,* for we have a built-in tendency to repress unpleasant, painful, or embarrassing emotions. These repressed feelings are the stimulus for TMS and other disorders like it. Anxiety and anger are two of those undesirable emotions that we would rather not be aware of, and so the mind keeps them in the subterranean precincts of the subconscious if it possibly can. All of this is discussed in detail in the psychology chapter. (See page 34.)

Then there's the person who says, "There was absolutely nothing going on in my life when this began." But when we begin to discuss the trials and tribulations of daily life, it is usually clear that this person is generating anxiety all the time. I think there is a gradual buildup in such people until a threshold is reached, at which point the symptoms begin. Once it is pointed out to them, these patients have little trouble recognizing that they are the kind of perfectionist, highly responsible people who generate a lot of subconscious anger and anxiety in response to the pressures of everyday life.

The Delayed-Onset Reaction

There is another interesting pattern that we see very often. In these cases, patients go through a highly stressful period that may last for weeks or months, such as an illness in the family or a financial crisis. They are physically fine as they live through the trouble, but one or two weeks after it's all over, they have an attack of back pain, either acute or slow onset. It seems as though they rise to the occasion and do whatever they have to do to deal with the trouble, but once it's over, the accumulated anxiety threatens to overwhelm them, and so the pain begins.

Another way of looking at it is that they don't have time to be sick during the crisis; all of their emotional energy goes into coping with the trouble.

A third possibility is that the crisis or stressful situation is providing enough emotional pain and distraction that a physical pain isn't necessary. The pain syndrome seems to function to divert the person's attention away from repressed undesirable emotions like anxiety and anger. When one is living through a crisis, there is more than enough unpleasantness going on and one has no need for a distraction.

Whatever the psychological explanation, this is a common pattern and it is important to recognize it so that the back pain will not be blamed on some "physical" condition.

The Weekend-Vacation Syndrome

When we generate anxiety depends mostly on the details of our personality structure. Not uncommonly, people will report that they almost always have an attack of pain when they are on vacation, or if they already have pain that it gets worse on weekends. For some the reason is obvious. They are very anxious about their work or business when they are away from it. It's a bit like the delayed reaction; as long as they are on the job, they may be "burning up" the anxiety, but when they are away from it, supposedly relaxing, the anxiety accumulates.

Speaking of relaxing, one often hears the advice "Relax," as though that's something one can do voluntarily. There are also numerous techniques around for promoting relaxation, like drugs, meditation, and biofeedback, to name a few. However, unless the relaxation process succeeds in reducing repressed anxiety and anger, people will develop things like TMS and tension headaches despite the attempt to induce relaxation. Some people don't know how to leave their daily concerns behind them and shift attention to something pleasurable. I remember a patient who said that her pain would invariably begin when she got herself a drink and sat down to relax.

Recently I saw a young man who illustrated the vacation syndrome very well. He described having been under a lot of stress for a long time, but without any back pain. It wasn't until he was on his honeymoon that he was awakened one night with a "nightmarish dream" followed immediately by a severe back spasm in which, he said, "my back went completely out." Of course, it might have been due to the stresses and strains of being newly married,

22

but he was an extremely conscientious type, and I was inclined to connect it with his work.

He was still having symptoms when I saw him three months later, no doubt due to the fact that an MRI had shown a disc herniation at the lower end of the spine and the possibility of surgery had been discussed. (An MRI, or magnetic resonance imaging, is an advanced diagnostic procedure that is capable of producing an image of body soft tissues, allowing one to detect the presence of such things as tumors or herniated discs.)

However, he read my book on TMS, thought that he was typical of the patients described, and came in to see me. The examination was conclusive for TMS. In fact, it showed that his symptoms could not be due to the herniated disc, for he had weakness in two sets of muscles in his leg, something that the herniated disc could not have caused. Only involvement of the sciatic nerve, as is typical in TMS, could have produced this neurological picture. At any rate, he was delighted to learn that TMS was the basis for his back troubles and had a rapid recovery.

Another explanation, often difficult for people to admit to themselves, is that there are great sources of anxiety and anger in their personal lives, like a bad marriage, trouble with children, having to care for an elderly parent. We have seen numerous examples of this: women trapped in bad marriages that they cannot stand and yet are unable to break out of because of their emotional and/or financial dependence on their husbands; people who feel perfectly competent at what they do for a living but who cannot deal with a difficult spouse or child.

I recall a woman with a persistent pain problem who lived with a very difficult brother. Despite psychotherapy, the pain continued. One day she told me that she had done a very unusual thing; she had gotten furious at her brother, had shouted and ranted at him and stormed out of the house. And with that—the pain disappeared. Unfortunately, she could not maintain her strong posture and the pain returned.

The Holiday Syndrome

One often hears or reads that holidays may be stressful. What should be a time of relaxation and fun often turns out to be unpleasant for some people. I have been struck by the fact that many patients will report the onset of attacks of TMS before, during, or shortly after major holidays.

The reason is obvious: Big holidays usually mean a lot of work, particularly for women, who take the responsibility in our culture for organizing and carrying out the festivities. And, of course, society demands that this be done cheerfully, with a smile. Usually the women are completely unaware that they are generating great quantities of resentment, and the onset of pain comes as a complete surprise.

THE NATURAL HISTORY OF TMS

What are the common patterns of TMS? What happens over time if one continues to be plagued by this disorder?

Conditioning

Essential to an understanding of this subject is knowledge about a very important phenomenon known as *conditioning*. A more modern term meaning the same thing is *programming*. All animals, including humans, are conditionable. The phenomenon is best known by the experiment reported by the Russian physiologist Pavlov, who is credited with the discovery of conditioning. His experiment demonstrated that animals develop associations that can produce automatic and reproducible physical reactions. In the research study, he rang a bell each time he fed a group of dogs. After repeating this a few times, he found that the dogs would salivate if he rang the bell even without the presentation of food. They had become conditioned to have a physical reaction at the sound of the bell.

The process of conditioning, or programming, seems to be very important in determining when the person with TMS will have pain. For example, a common complaint of people with low back pain is that it is invariably brought on by sitting. This is such a benign activity one is mystified by the fact that it initiates pain. But conditioning occurs when two things go on simultaneously, so it is easy to imagine that at some point early in the course of the TMS experience, the person happens to be having pain while sitting. The brain makes the association between sitting and the presence of pain, and that person is now programmed to expect pain with sitting. In other words, the pain occurs because of its subconscious association with sitting, not because sitting is bad for the back. That is one way a conditioned response may be established. There must be others I am unaware of, since sitting is such a common problem for people with low back pain. Car seats have a bad reputation, so a person expects to have pain when he or she gets into a car.

Often people are programmed to have pain because of things they have heard or been told by a practitioner. "Never bend at the waist" means the onset of pain is a sure thing when they bend from then on, although it may never have caused pain before. Someone says that sitting compresses the lower end of the spine—so, of course, it's got to hurt when you sit. Standing in one place, lifting, carrying—all have a bad reputation and will quickly be conditioned into a patient's pattern.

Many people report that the pain is relieved by walking; others say that walking brings it on. Some have a great deal of pain at night and cannot sleep. One man worked hard all day long with a fair amount of heavy lifting and never a twinge of pain. Every night he would wake up about 3:00 A.M. with severe pain that persisted until he got out of bed. Clearly a conditioned reaction.

Others report that they sleep well but develop pain as soon as they wake up and get out of bed. In these patients, the pain usually increases in severity as the day goes on.

Based on history and physical examination, all of these

people have TMS but are programmed to believe they suffer from something else. What gives strong support to the idea that these reactions are conditioned is that they disappear within a few weeks as patients go through my treatment program. If they were structurally based, they would not go away after treatment (consisting primarily of lecture seminars), which is what happens with successfully treated patients. The conditioning is broken by the educational process.

One cannot overemphasize the importance of conditioning in TMS, for it explains many of the reactions that patients don't understand. If someone says, "I can lift a very light weight but anything over five pounds will cause pain," the pain can't be based on structural grounds. Or this example: a woman who could bend over and touch her palms to the floor without pain but told me she always felt pain when she put her shoes on!

Many of these conditioned responses stem from the fear that people develop when they have back pain, especially in the low back. They have been told and they have read that the back is fragile, vulnerable and easily injured, so if they try to do something vigorous, like jog or swim or vacuum the floor, their backs begin to hurt. They have learned to associate activity with pain; they expect it, so it happens. That is conditioning.

The specific posture or activity that brings on the pain is not important per se. What is essential is to know that it has been programmed in as a part of the TMS and is therefore of psychological rather than physical significance.

Common Patterns of TMS

Perhaps the most common pattern is for the person to have *recurrent acute attacks* of the kind described earlier. These may last from days to weeks or even months, with the most acute pain subsiding after a few days. They are traditionally treated with bed rest, painkillers, and anti-inflammatory drugs, administered by mouth or by injection. If the patient is hospitalized, traction is often employed, though its purpose is to immobilize the patient and not to pull the spinal bones apart, since this could not be done with the weights used. I do not instruct my patients what to do for an acute attack, for it is the goal of this program to see that the attacks don't occur—to prevent them. However, occasionally I am called upon to advise someone having an acute attack; as stated earlier in the chapter, it's essentially a question of waiting it out. I may prescribe a strong painkiller but not an anti-inflammatory drug, since there is no inflammation.

The irony of the usual experience with one of these attacks is that most patients would be better off if they consulted no one. This is unwise, however, because every once in a while, there may be something physiologically important going on, and so one must be examined by a physician. Assuming nothing truly serious, like a tumor, is present, the usual diagnosis is some spinal structural abnormality. A scary diagnosis (degenerative disc disease, herniated disc, arthritis, spinal stenosis, or facet syndrome) plus the dire warnings of what will happen if the patient doesn't take sufficient bed rest and cautioning about never again jogging or using a vacuum cleaner or bowling or playing tennis is the perfect combination for multiplied and persistent pain.

But the human spirit is more or less indomitable, and eventually the symptoms fade, leaving someone who is essentially free of pain but permanently scarred, not physically but emotionally. Except for the very brave few, most people who have had such an attack never again engage in vigorous physical activity with an easy mind. They have been sensitized by the experience and all that it is supposed to imply, and they see themselves, to a greater or lesser degree, as permanently altered. They fear another attack and eventually it comes. It may be six months or a year later, but the prophecy is fulfilled and the dreaded event occurs again. As before, the person usually attributes the attack to some physical incident. This time there may be leg pain as well as back pain, and now there is talk of surgery should a herniated disc be found on MRI or CT scan. (CT, or computed tomography, is an advanced X-ray technique that can, like the MRI, give information about soft tissues as well as bone.) This further increases anxiety, and the pain may become even more severe.

This pattern of recurrence of acute attacks is very common. As time goes on, the attacks tend to come more frequently, to be more severe and to last longer. And with each new attack, the fear increases and there is an increased tendency to limit physical activities. Some patients become virtually disabled as time goes on.

In my view, physical restrictions and the fear of physical activity represent the worst aspect of these pain syndromes. They are ever present, though the pain may come and go. They have a profound effect on all aspects of life: work, family, leisure time. Indeed, I have known patients with TMS who were much more disabled in terms of their daily lives than patients who were paralyzed in both legs. Many of the latter go to work every day on their own, raise families, and in every way lead normal lives, except that they are in wheelchairs. The severe TMS patient may have to stay in bed most of the day because of the pain.

Eventually most people who have recurrent attacks will develop a *chronic pattern*. They will begin to have some pain all the time, usually mild, but exacerbated by a variety of activities or postures to which they have become conditioned. "I can lie on my left side but not on my right"; "I must always have a pillow between my knees in bed"; "I never go anywhere without my seat cushion"; "My body corset (or neck collar) is absolutely essential if I am to remain free of pain"; "If I sit for more than five minutes, I get severe pain"; "The only chair I can sit on has to have a hard seat and a straight back"; and on and on.

And to some the pain becomes the primary focus of their lives. It is not uncommon to hear people say that the pain is the first thing they are aware of when they awaken in the morning and the last thing they think about when they go to sleep. They become obsessed with it.

There is great variety in the manifestations of TMS. There are those who have a little pain all the time with varying degrees of physical restriction. Others have occasional acute attacks but live essentially normal lives in between with little or no restriction.

What I have been describing are the more common manifestations of TMS and the most dramatic, those in the low back and legs. However, a severe episode involving the neck, shoulders, and arms can be very dramatic too—and just as physically restricting. Here is a typical example.

The patient was a middle-aged man who had been having recurrent attacks of pain in the neck and shoulders and pain, numbness, and tingling in his hands for about three years prior to the time I saw him. The episode that brought him to me had begun about eight months previously with pain in the left arm. He saw two neurologists, had a variety of sophisticated tests, and was told that the pain was the result of a "disc problem" in the neck. There was debate whether he should have immediate surgery; he was warned that he might become paralyzed if he didn't. Not surprisingly, the pain spread from his arm to his neck and back; he was unable to ski or play tennis, two of his favorite sports. He was very frightened.

My examination disclosed that he had TMS and that there were no neurological abnormalities. Fortunately, a third neurologist concluded that there was no structural basis for his pain, so he was able to accept the diagnosis of TMS with an easy mind. He went through the program and in a few weeks was free of pain and able to resume his usual athletic activities. He has not had a recurrence.

Sometimes the shoulder is the site of the trouble or the knee. To anyone who tries to be physically active, knee pain can be very debilitating. I have had such an episode and can attest to the fact that it can be scary, persistent, and restricting. Any of the tendons and ligaments in the arms and legs and any of the muscles and nerves of the neck, shoulders, back, and buttocks can be involved in TMS.

Though we must identify the structures involved in each case, this is the least important part of the consultation. Each encounter with a patient is an excursion into that person's life. After we have established which body parts are involved, that information must be put aside, for we do not work on the muscles, nerves, and ligaments directly. Something in that person's emotional life that might have played a role in producing the symptoms must be addressed.

There comes to mind the case of a man who had found himself financially well-off enough to retire from business at an early age and who shortly thereafter developed the pain syndrome for which I saw him. As we talked, it became apparent that since his retirement, he had become preoccupied with a number of family problems, there had been a number of deaths in the family, he was worried about the health of the business he had left (in the hands of relatives), and he had begun to wonder what his life was all about now that he was retired and was thinking about aging and mortality for the first time. His concern about these matters, considered consciously and unconsciously, had produced sufficient anxiety (and anger) to precipitate the TMS. Conventional medicine had attributed his pain to an aging spine, and treatment for that had, naturally, failed. He had TMS; his troubles were not in his spine—they were in his life.

To summarize, TMS may involve postural muscles, nerves that are in and around those muscles, and a variety of tendons and ligaments in the arms and legs. In the areas involved, the patient has pain, possibly feelings of pins and needles and/or weakness. There are many different patterns and locations of symptoms and considerable variation in severity, ranging from mild annoyance to almost total disability.

Recurrent attacks, fear of recurrence and physical activity, and failure to find successful treatment characterize TMS.

The symptoms of pain, numbness, tingling, and weakness are intended by the brain to suggest that something is physically wrong. To most people, practitioners and laymen alike, "physically wrong" means injury, weakness, incompetence, and degeneration, singly or in combination. To further this view of the symptoms, the pain often begins in association with some physical activity, the more vigorous the better. The patient can't help but conclude that something has been injured or displaced. "My back went out" is a common description of the event.

Also very important to advancing the idea of structural incompetence is the powerful tendency for people to become programmed to fear a variety of simple, common things like sitting, standing in one place, bending, and lifting.

The net effect of symptoms, fears, and alterations in lifestyle and daily activities is to produce someone whose attention is strongly focused on the body. As shall be seen in succeeding chapters, that is the purpose of the syndrome—to create a distraction so that undesirable emotions can be avoided. It seems a heavy price to pay, but then the inner workings of the mind are not really known, and we can only suspect its deep aversion to frightening, painful feelings.

2

The Psychology
of TMS

Neck, shoulder, and back pain syndromes are not mechanical problems to be cured by mechanical means. They have to do with people's feelings, their personalities, and the vicissitudes of life. If this is true, the conventional management of these pain syndromes is a medical travesty. Traditional medical diagnoses focus on the machine, the body, while the real problem seems to relate to what makes the machine work—the mind. TMS is characterized by physical pain, but that acute discomfort is induced by psychological phenomena rather than structural abnormalities or muscle deficiency. This is an exceedingly important point, and just how this works will be clarified in the pages to follow. But first a few definitions to be sure that the terms are clear.

TENSION

Tension is a word that is widely used and means different things to different people; in my work and in this book, the disorder is called the Tension Myositis Syndrome. The word *tension* is used here to refer to emotions that are generated in the unconscious mind and that, to a large extent, remain there. These feelings are the result of a complicated interaction between different parts of our minds and between the mind and the outside world. Many of them are either unpleasant, painful, or embarrassing, in some way unacceptable to us and/or society, and so we *repress* them. The kinds of feelings referred to are anxiety, anger, and low self-esteem (feelings of inferiority). They are repressed because the mind doesn't want us to experience them, nor does it want them to be seen by the outside world. It is likely that, if given a conscious choice, most of us would decide to deal with the bad feelings; but as the human mind is presently constituted, they are immediately and automatically repressed—one has no choice.

To sum up, the word *tension* will be used here to refer to repressed, unacceptable emotions.

STRESS

The word *stress* is often confused with tension and seems to stand for anything that is emotionally negative. I like to use it to refer to any factor, influence, or condition that tests, strains, or in any way puts pressure on the individual. We can be stressed physically or emotionally. Excessive heat and cold are physical stressors; a demanding job and family problems are emotional ones. The stress involved in TMS leads to emotional reactions that are repressed.

The work of Dr. Hans Selye is credited with first drawing attention to how stress affects the body; his research and writing were prolific and stand as one of the major accomplishments of medicine in the twentieth century. Dr. Selye's definition of *biological stress* is "the nonspecific response of the body to any demand made upon it."

Stress can be either external or internal to the individual. Examples of external stress are your job, financial problems, illness, change of job or home, caring for children or parents. However, the internal stressors appear to be more important in the production of tension. These are one's own personality attributes, like conscientiousness, perfectionism, the need to excel, and so forth. People often say that they have a very stressful job and that's why they're tense. But if they weren't conscientious about doing a good job, if they weren't trying to succeed, achieve, and excel, they wouldn't generate tension. Often such people are highly competitive and determined to get ahead. Typically, they are more critical of themselves than others are of them.

A homemaker and mother with a similar personality stresses herself in the same way as someone in the work world, but the focus of her concerns is the family. She worries about her children, her husband, her parents. She wants the best for everyone and will do everything in her power to bring it about. She may also tell you that it is important to her that everyone like her, that she gets very upset if she feels that anyone is displeased with her. (This compulsion to please is, of course, not limited to women; a middle-aged man expressed identical sentiments in my office recently.)

Stress, then, is outside what one might call the inner

core of the emotional structure and is composed of the stresses and strains of daily life and, more importantly, aspects of one's own personality. And stress leads to tension (repressed, unacceptable feelings). Now let's take a closer look at the personality.

THE CONSCIOUS MIND

The part of your personality that you're aware of resides in the conscious mind; it is the realm of emotions you can feel. You feel sad, glad, exhilarated, depressed; you also know that you are conscientious, hardworking, a worrier, perhaps compulsive and perfectionistic. You may realize that you are often irritable or you're aware of having a need to assert yourself. A man may have strong feelings of masculine superiority and be aware of it, indeed proud of it. These make up the conscious mind, and they seem to determine what we do in life and how we conduct ourselves. But do they? Often these outward characteristics reflect inner drives of which we may be totally unaware, so it is important to look at the subconscious mind, as we shall do in a moment.

Many people with TMS are aware of possessing conscientious personality characteristics. They often refer to themselves as Type A people, after the work of Dr. Meyer Friedman and Dr. Ray Rosenman, who described the type of person prone to coronary artery disease in their book *Type A Behavior and Your Heart* (New York: Alfred A. Knopf, 1974). What they described is someone who is hard-driving, obsessed with work to the extreme. Such a person might claim to work eighteen hours a day and never feel tired.

This is not characteristic of someone who gets TMS. Though hardworking, there is awareness of one's limitations and certainly some awareness of oneself as an emotional being. I have the impression that the true Type A person is not at all in touch with himself emotionally. He or she tends to deny feelings as though they are a sign of weakness. That there is an important difference between the patient who gets TMS and the Type A person is based on the observation that it is rare for TMS patients to have a history of coronary artery disease or to develop it later. There have been a few, of course, but nothing like the numbers of patients who have had other things, like stomach trouble, colitis, hay fever, tension headache, migraine headache, acne, hives, and many other conditions that seem to be related to tension. These appear to be equivalents of TMS and reflect a lower level of compulsivity than that of the Type A person.

The personality characteristics of which we are aware represent only a part of our emotional makeup and may be less important than that which is unconscious.

THE UNCONSCIOUS MIND

The word *unconscious* has an unfortunate other use—that is, to be out of contact as in sleep or when brain damaged. However, it is firmly entrenched in the psychological literature as referring to that part of emotional activity of which we are usually unaware, and we should, therefore, use the word when discussing emotions. We would probably be more comfortable with the word *subconscious* and will use it when talking about things below the level of awareness other than the emotions.

The unconscious is subterranean, the realm of the hidden and mysterious and the place where all sorts of feelings may reside, not all logical, not all nice, and some of them downright scary. We get some hint of the kind of things that inhabit the unconscious from our dreams. Someone said that every night when we go to sleep, we all go quietly and safely insane, because that's when the remnants of childish, primitive, wild behaviors that are a part of everyone's emotional repertoire can show themselves without being monitored by the waking, conscious mind. The unconscious is the repository of all of our feelings, regardless of their social or personal acceptability. To know about the unconscious is extremely important, for what goes on down there may be responsible for those personality characteristics that drive us to behave as we do when we're awake—and the unconscious is where TMS and other disorders like it originate.

It is an interesting fact that the overwhelming majority of emotional and mental activity occurs below the level of consciousness. The human mind is something like an iceberg—the part that we are aware of, the conscious mind, represents a very small part of the total. It is in the subconscious mind that all of the complicated processing goes on that allows us, for example, to generate written and oral language; to think, to reason, to remember; in short, to do most of the things that identify us as human beings. Our ability to make sense of the things we see, to recognize faces, and dozens of other mental activities we take for granted are the result of brain activity of which we are unaware.

It is likely that the majority of emotional reactions occur in the unconscious. Feelings that remain there do so because they are repressed, and it is these that are responsible for the sequence of events that cause TMS. This condition begins and ends in the unconscious.

Incidentally, one should make a distinction, as Freud did a long time ago, between mental items that are not conscious but that can be brought to consciousness with effort, like the things in our memories—Freud called that mental domain the *preconscious*—and things in the unconscious that are unavailable and cannot be recalled. We simply don't know they are there.

To better understand how and why TMS gets started, it's essential to look at some of these unconscious emotional processes.

Low Self-Esteem

I find it almost shocking to realize how common it is for people to have feelings of inferiority deep inside. There must be a cultural reason for this that is reflected in the way we are managed as children and therefore the way we develop. This is a subject that should be studied intensively and no doubt will be someday. These feelings of inferiority are deep and hidden but reveal themselves through our behavior. We generally overcompensate for bad feelings, so if we feel weak, we act strong. This was beautifully illustrated many years ago when a self-proclaimed "tough guy" came under my care for crippling back pain. The staff reported that he was constantly bragging about his prowess in hand-to-hand combat, in financial matters, and with women. In my office, he wept inconsolably about his inability to cope with his back pain. Emotionally, he was a very little boy trying desperately to prove to himself and the world how tough he was.

It is likely that for most of us, the compulsive need to do well, succeed, and achieve is a reflection of deep-seated feelings of inferiority. Wherever it comes from, the need to accomplish or live up to some ideal role, such as being the best parent, student, or worker, is very common in people who get TMS.

A typical example was a patient who through compulsive hard work established a very successful business and became the patriarch and benefactor of his large family. He enjoyed the role but felt the responsibility deeply. Throughout his entire adult life, he had low back pain, which resisted all attempts at treatment. By the time I saw him, the pain patterns were deeply ingrained and part of his everyday life. He understood the concept of tension-induced pain but was unable to erase the patterns of a lifetime. He felt that he was too old to engage in psychotherapy, which is often required for patients like this. The primary benefit he derived from treatment was the reassurance that there was nothing structurally wrong with his back.

Another patient was a young man in his twenties who had his first child shortly before he opened a new branch of the family business. The simultaneous imposition of these new responsibilities in this very conscientious young man induced severe low back pain due to TMS. As soon as he became aware that the source of his symptoms was inner tension, the pain disappeared. As will be seen later, awareness is the key to recovery from TMS.

What these two people had in common was a great sense of responsibility and a strong inner drive to succeed in both business and family matters. Such people don't need to be monitored; they are self-motivated, self-disciplined, their own severest critics.

People who get TMS are often intensely competitive, success oriented, achieving, and usually very accomplished. In our culture, success often requires the ability to compete effectively, and they do. They are accustomed to putting a great deal of pressure on themselves and often feel as though they have not done enough.

Sometimes the perfectionism manifests itself in unusual ways. I remember seeing a young man once who had grown up on a farm. He said that when he had read my first book, he didn't see how this perfectionism applied to him until he realized that at haying time he had a powerful compulsion to stack the bales of hay perfectly.

At this point, if you're mentally scratching your head and wondering why being hardworking, conscientious, or compulsive and perfectionistic should bring on TMS, you're right. It is clear that there is a relationship between these personality characteristics and this pain syndrome, but what is it? To understand this, we need to think about anxiety and anger.

Anxiety and Anger

Not being trained in psychology or psychiatry, I am aware that my concepts and explanations of what goes on in this psychophysiologic process may sound naive to professionals in these fields. However, this is a book for the general public, and the lack of jargon and complex concepts will probably be welcome. My lack of training in these fields notwithstanding, what I have observed about the nature of this pain syndrome and its causes should be taken seriously by psychology professionals. We are dealing here with the almost totally unexplored territory between what is purely mental-emotional and what is physical. There is a powerful and important link that, sadly, contemporary medical science (with a few notable exceptions) is unwilling to explore. The reason for that reluctance is discussed in chapter 7, "Mind and Body." My experience in the diagnosis and treatment of TMS throws some light on what is going on in that mysterious domain where the emotional and the physical connect.

Anger and anxiety are discussed together, for I think they are closely related and are the primary repressed feelings behind TMS and other disorders like it.

It was obvious from the beginning of my experience with TMS that most patients shared the personality characteristics described above. Those who denied possessing any of those characteristics eventually admitted that they had many emotional concerns, but they tended to deny them and instead would "put them out of my mind."

With this repertoire of personality traits, it was not difficult to postulate that anxiety was responsible for TMS, since such an individual would be anxious about how things would turn out. Anxiety is a uniquely human phenomenon, closely related to fear but much more sophisticated, for it is rooted in a capacity animals do not possess—the ability to anticipate. Anxiety arises in response to the perception of danger and is logical unless the perception is illogical, as is often the case. The anxious person tends to anticipate danger, often where there is little or none. This is the nature of the human animal. However, he or she is often not aware of this anxiety, for it is generated in the unconscious out of feelings that are largely unconscious and are kept in the unconscious through the well-known mechanism of *repression*. Because of the unpleasant, embarrassing, often painful nature of these feelings and the anxiety they generate, there is a strong need to keep them out of consciousness, which is the purpose of repression. As will be seen later, the purpose of TMS is to assist in the process of repression.

Narcissism

The role of low self-esteem was described above. Standing right beside this deeply buried feeling is another of equal importance, called *narcissism*. It refers to the human tendency to love oneself—that is, to be self-centered to an excessive degree. The evolution of culture in the United States seems to have produced people who are much more "I" than "we" oriented. I have heard it said that many of the American Indian languages had no pronouns for *I* and *me* because of a powerful sense of community and of being part of something larger than themselves. By contrast, contemporary North Americans believe in individualism and have great admiration for the person who "goes it alone." But the other side of that coin is that the individual may become overly focused on himself and, if he is not motivated by lofty ideals, tend to greediness and avarice. It is shocking and revealing to contemplate respected members of the business community or government engaged in felonious acts, but it is not surprising when one considers that this is a logical extension of today's narcissistic trends.

Anger

Narcissism exists in all human beings to some degree. When it is strong, it can make trouble since it means that the person is easily irritated, often frustrated by contact with others who do not do his bidding or do it badly. The result is anger, and if the person is very narcissistic, he or she may be angry all the time but never know it because, like anxiety, it has been repressed. It's all there in the unconscious mind.

Here's a seeming paradox. On the one hand, we have poor self-esteem, but then our narcissism leads us to behave emotionally like reigning monarchs. It is the story of the prince and the pauper—they are one and the same person. These diametrically different feelings are opposite sides of the same coin, though it may strike us as strange that they generally exist simultaneously.

How typical of the human mind. It appears to be a storehouse of often conflicting feelings and tendencies, most of which we are totally unaware of.

We are angry for other reasons. In fact, anything that makes us anxious (all unconscious) will tend to make us angry as well. You're trying to do a good job; you hope it turns out well (anxious), but you're also resentful of the problems with which you must contend, like other people and their needs (angry).

Although the production of anxiety and anger is often work related, personal relationships are an equally common source of repressed emotions. Family dynamics often produce serious problems that may be unrecognized because of their subtlety.

One of my patients was a woman in her late forties who had had a sheltered adolescence, an early marriage, and, as dictated by her culture, thereafter had devoted herself exclusively to home and family. She did an excellent job since she was an intelligent, competent, and compassionate woman. However, there came a time when she began to resent the fact that she had not been allowed to go to school as a child and could not read and write, could not drive a car, and had been denied many experiences because the needs of her family so dominated her life. She was totally unaware of the existence of this resentment and, as a consequence, developed a long, disabling history of back pain, including unsuccessful surgery. When she came to my attention, she was in constant pain and was almost totally unable to function. Through the education program and psychotherapy, she became aware of these repressed feelings and the pain gradually disappeared.

The process was not without psychological trauma, for now she was faced with the disapproval of her family and friends and her own deeply ingrained attitudes. She was in considerable conflict and now experienced emotional pain. But this was appropriate and vastly preferable to the physical pain, of which she had been a helpless victim.

An important source of anger and resentment, of which we are usually unaware, stems from our sense of responsibility to those who are close to us, like parents, spouses, and children. Though we love them, they may burden us in many ways and the resultant anger is internalized. How can one be angry at elderly parents or a baby?

A good example: A man in his forties went to visit his elderly parents in another city. Before the weekend was over, he had a recurrence of back pain, the first since successfully completing the TMS therapeutic program a year before. When I suggested that the return of pain meant that something was bothering him subconsciously, he said the weekend had been pleasant. But then he revealed that his mother was feeble, that he had spent most of the weekend ministering to her needs, and that both of his parents were a worry to him. To make matters worse, they lived a plane ride away. But he was a good man, and his parents couldn't help it if they were getting old. So his *natural* (intrinsic, unconscious, narcissistically inspired) *annoyance* (anger, resentment) was completely repressed and, for reasons that shall be clarified shortly, gave rise to the recurrence of back pain.

Or take the case of the young father whose firstborn turns out to be a nonsleeper. Not only does he lose sleep but also his wife is pretty much tied up with baby around the clock. He has to pitch in during his free time, their social life is much curtailed, and what was a long honeymoon before baby came is now a grind. He develops back pain because he's mad at the baby (ridiculous) and is angry at his wife because she can no longer minister to his emotional and physical needs as she had before (absurd). And to make matters worse, he has become a part-time nursemaid and cook. But he doesn't know about any of these feelings—they are deeply buried in his unconscious, and to make sure they stay there, he gets back pain—TMS.

There is a large group of psychologists and doctors who would put a different interpretation on the young father's plight. They would say his back hurts from lifting the baby and not getting enough sleep and that the pain is very bad because he's trying to get out of doing his part with the baby—now he has a good excuse. Of course, they say, this is all subconscious.

This is the so-called secondary gain theory of chronic pain. The trouble with it is that it presupposes a structural reason for the pain, which is usually untenable (this baby's father played high school and college football), and, secondly, it elevates to preeminence a feeling that is either minor or nonexistent, that the person is deriving some benefit from the pain. Behavioral psychologists like it, however, because it's simple, and all you have to do is reward "nonpain behavior" and punish its opposite. There is no getting involved with messy unconscious feelings like anxiety and anger. Years ago, before I knew about TMS, I tried this approach and found it singularly ineffective. Little wonder—it was the wrong diagnosis.

All family relationships are emotionally loaded. It is one of the first things to be considered when someone has an attack of TMS that seems to come out of nowhere. The combination of real concern and love for the family member and inner resentment of the duties and responsibilities associated with the relationship is a source of deep conflict, the stuff of which TMS is made.

Here is a classic story with some interesting sidelights about the natural history of TMS. The patient was a thirty-nine-year-old married man who ran a family business originally started by his father. He told me that his father was still active in the business but that he had become a hindrance rather than a help. He admitted to conflict with his father over this and to feeling guilty about the whole thing. The pain syndrome had begun about two and a half years before, and about four months into the experience, he read my first book. He decided it was hogwash and proceeded to make his way through the medical system, determined to get rid of the pain. He said he saw many doctors and tried virtually every available treatment, with no success. Two years later, he was still in pain, was rapidly becoming obsessed with it, and was extremely limited physically. He was afraid of any physical activity and could not even bend. At that point, he read the book again and reported with incredulity, "It had a totally different effect on me." He said he saw himself on every page. His explanation was that he had to go through all the tests and doctors before he was ready to acknowledge a psychological basis for the pain.

Needless to say, he did very well on the program and was soon free of pain. During the consultation, I found him to be so perceptive and psychologically attuned I could not imagine that he had originally rejected the diagnosis. It was a lesson to me: One of the unfortunate realities about working with a disorder like TMS is that most people will reject the idea until they are desperate for a solution.

The reason for the pain syndrome, the man's conflict over his relationship with his father, was very clear.

Here is another good example of the role of family dynamics in producing symptoms. A woman who had been successfully treated for low back pain two years prior called one day to tell me that she had now developed neck, shoulder, and arm pain but was certain it was due to a painful psychological situation involving her husband and teenage stepdaughter. I encouraged her to carry on without formal treatment, but the situation remained unresolved and the pain became increasingly severe; she also lost considerable motion in both shoulders, a common consequence of TMS in the neck and shoulders. Then one day she decided to face the problem squarely and confront her husband. The result was a surprisingly easy solution that defused the entire situation, and with resolution of her personal problems, the pain disappeared. She had undoubtedly harbored great resentment, and as long as she did, the pain persisted. I shall have more to say about how one deals with this kind of situation in the treatment chapter, but this case clearly illustrates the relationship between repressed anger and TMS.

One of the great sources of conflict in the unconscious is the battle that rages between those feelings and needs that stem from the narcissistic impulses described above and another very real part of the mind that is concerned with what is appropriate, reasonable, and mature or, even more demanding, what you should be doing. The well-known psychoanalyst, writer, and teacher Karen Horney described what she called "the tyranny of the should," which may dominate someone's life. Patients often describe in detail how their lives are governed by these behavioral imperatives. One woman told me, after denying that she was compulsive or perfectionistic, that she came from a family that prided itself on its strength of character and rigidity—"stiff upper lip" and all that stuff. It was clear that there were other parts of her personality that were softer and more pliable, so the conflict in her unconscious must have been considerable.

Sometimes the pressure to behave in a certain way comes from one's culture. I recall a strikingly attractive woman who was part of a religious group that believed in very large families; six or eight children were not unusual. Though she acknowledged that her pain was due to "tension," it persisted and she couldn't understand why. I suggested that she might be resentful of the work and responsibility for such a large family. For a long time she denied this, insisting that she felt no such resentment, and the pain continued, sometimes very severely. I pointed out that she would not be aware of the feeling since it was unconscious and repressed. Perseverance, both hers and mine, paid off. She began to get inklings of her deeply repressed resentment, and then had a dramatic resolution of her symptoms.

The longer I work with TMS, the more impressed I am with the role of anger. We have all learned to repress it so completely that we are totally unaware of its existence in many situations. In fact, I have begun to wonder if anger is not more fundamental to the development of symptoms than anxiety and, indeed, whether anxiety itself may be a reaction to repressed anger.

The following story made a deep impression on me. The man was in his midforties and, among other things, had a history of having occasional panic attacks. These represent acute anxiety. After having examined him and established that he had TMS, we discussed the psychology of the disorder, and I told him that I was beginning to suspect that anger might be more important than anxiety. He said that something had just happened to him that supported that supposition. He had become extremely angry at someone and was at the point of starting an altercation when he decided that it would not be appropriate, that he had better swallow it. Within moments, he had a panic attack! He was probably more than angry—he was in a rage, and the need to repress it, both unconsciously and consciously, necessitated some kind of reaction, hence the panic attack. As we shall see in a moment, this is precisely the kind of situation that brings on TMS and other physical reactions. But first let's consider the phenomenon of repression. Where does it come from?

Repression

I remember a mother telling me proudly how she had stopped the temper tantrums in her little fifteen-month-old. The "wise" family doctor suggested that she splash ice water in the child's face when he started to have a tantrum. It worked beautifully—he never had another tantrum. At the ripe age of fifteen months, he had learned the technique of repression. He had been programmed to repress anger, because it produced very unpleasant consequences, and he would carry that dubious talent with him throughout his life. Now when confronted with the multitude of frustrating, annoying, sometimes enraging things that happen to people every day, this man automatically internalizes his natural anger, and when that anger collects and builds up, he will have TMS or some such physical reaction in response to it.

The story illustrates one of the sources of the need to repress: innocent parental influence. This may be the most common reason for learning to repress. In an attempt to make good people of their children, parents may inadvertently induce the conditions for psychological difficulty later in life.

When you think about it, there are many reasons why we repress anger, all logical and mostly unconscious. Everyone wants to be liked or loved; no one enjoys disapproval, so we repress unlovable behavior. We would hate to admit it, but unconsciously we fear reprisal. The cultural imperatives of family and society provide strong motivation not to show anger; this becomes deeply imbedded, starting as it does in early childhood. We realize, all unconsciously, that anger is often inappropriate, springing from irritants that ought not make us angry, and so we repress. Instinctively we feel that anger is demeaning, and perhaps even more powerful, we feel a loss of control when we are angry, and that is something the TMS personality finds hard to take. All of this is unconscious and thus we are unaware of our need to repress the anger. Instead we may experience a physical symptom, TMS or something gastrointestinal, for example.

I do that a lot. I have learned that heartburn means that I'm angry about something and don't know it. So I think about what might be causing the condition, and when I come up with the answer, the heartburn disappears. It is remarkable how well buried the anger usually is. Generally for me, it is something about which I am annoyed but have no idea how much it has angered me. Sometimes it is something that is so loaded emotionally, I don't come up with the answer for a long time.

After a seventeen-year experience working with TMS, it seems clear that, in our culture at least, we all generate anxiety and anger and that, in any culture, human beings repress potentially problematic emotions. Put another way, the psychological conditions that lead to psychophysiologic reactions like TMS, stomach ulcers, and colitis are universal; they only vary in degree. Those at the upper end of the severity spectrum, with more intense symptoms, we call *neurotic,* but in fact we are all more or less neurotic, making the term meaningless.

The concepts of repression and the unconscious are closely bound together. They were first put on a sound, scientific basis by Freud. There is a wonderful metaphor of the unconscious in Peter Gay's excellent biography of Freud, *Freud: A Life for Our Time* (New York: Norton, 1988), p. 128: "Rather, the unconscious proper resembles a maximum-security prison holding anti-social inmates languishing for years or recently arrived, inmates harshly treated and heavily guarded, but barely kept under control and *forever attempting to escape*" (italics added).

The emotional phenomena that have been described in this chapter are the "anti-social inmates" of the unconscious. We seem to have a built-in mechanism for avoiding what is emotionally unpleasant, which is the reason for repression. But there appears to be an equally strong force in the mind working to bring those feelings to consciousness ("forever attempting to escape"), and that is the reason for reinforcements, for what psychoanalysts call a *defense.*

A short time ago, I saw a woman who told the most interesting story. After I had examined her and told her she had TMS and what it meant, she said that the pain had begun after she invited an older sister to take a trip to Europe, at her expense. She began to worry about whether the sister would have a good time, felt that it was her responsibility to see that she did, and then got angry and resentful about having to feel that way. She further reported that she began to dream about her mother and sister and to recall her teenage resentments against them, based on the feeling (no doubt unjustified) that they "ganged up on her—to be good" and that she was excluded from their close relationship. All of this was enhanced by the fact that she felt her father, with whom she had been very close, had abandoned her—he died when she was eleven.

This is the kind of thing from which TMS often arises: anxiety, anger, resentment, with roots that go all the way back to childhood. I thought it remarkable of her to have come up with all that important psychological material with just a hint from me.

The universality of these psychological phenomena is supported by the strangely ignored fact that over 80 percent of the U.S. population has a history of these pain syndromes and that their incidence has increased geometrically over the last thirty years. Back and neck pain syndromes are the first cause of worker absenteeism in this country. It is estimated that somewhere around $56 billion are expended annually in the United States on the ravages of back pain. This virtual epidemic of pain syndromes can only be properly explained on the basis of a universal psychophysiological process.

PHYSICAL DEFENSES AGAINST REPRESSED EMOTIONS

For many years I was under the impression that TMS was a kind of physical expression or discharge of the repressed emotions just described. In fact, this is what I suggested in the first edition of this book. I had been aware since the early 1970s that these common back and neck pain syndromes were due to repressed emotions. Eighty-eight percent of a large group of patients with TMS had a history of other tension-related disorders, like stomach ulcers, colitis, tension headache, and migraine headache. But the idea of TMS as a physical manifestation of nervous tension was somehow unsatisfactory and incomplete. Most important, it did not explain the repeated observation that making a patient aware of the role of the pain as participant in a psychological process would lead to cessation of pain, to a "cure."

It was a psychoanalyst colleague, Dr. Stanley Coen, who suggested in the course of our working on a medical paper together that the role of the pain syndrome was not to express the hidden emotions but to prevent them from becoming conscious. This, he explained, is what is referred to as a *defense*. In other words, the pain of TMS (or the discomfort of a peptic ulcer, of colitis, of tension headache, or the terror of an asthmatic attack) is created in order to distract the attention of the sufferer from what is going on in the emotional sphere. It is intended to focus one's attention on the body instead of the mind. It is a response to the need to keep those terrible, antisocial, unkind, childish, angry, selfish feelings (the prisoners) from

56

becoming conscious. It follows from this that far from being a physical disorder in the usual sense, TMS is really part of a psychological process.

Defenses against repressed emotions work by diverting one's attention to something other than the emotions that are being kept hidden in the unconscious. Patients have different metaphors to describe the process: that the defense acts as a camouflage; that it is a diversion or distraction. To be successful, it must occupy one's attention, and it works even better if you are totally preoccupied or obsessed by whatever it is. That is why physical defenses are so good: They have the ability to really grab one's attention, particularly if they are painful, frightening, and disabling. This is exactly what happens with TMS.

The common back, neck, and shoulder pain syndromes have reached epidemic proportions in the United States over the past thirty years, because they have become the preferred defense against the repressed emotions described above. The mark of a good camouflage is that it will not be recognized for what it is, that no one will know that something is being hidden. Virtually no one suffering from them thinks that these pain syndromes are related to emotional factors. On the contrary, almost everyone thinks they are due to injury or a variety of congenital and degenerative abnormalities of the spine. There is another group of disorders that are part of the TMS repertoire and are thought to be due to soft tissue pathology (fibromyalgia, fibrositis, myofasciitis, among others), but these, too, are attributed to injury, muscle incompetence, and the like—the perfect camouflage. As long as the person's attention remains focused on the pain syndrome, there is no danger that the emotions will be revealed.

It has been a recurrent observation of mine that the more painful the repressed emotion, the more severe the pain of TMS has been. The patient who is found to be harboring enormous anger as a result of childhood abuses, for example, usually has severe, disabling pain, and the pain disappears only when that person has an opportunity to express the terrible, festering rage that has occupied his or her unconscious for years—another example of the potential of anger to initiate the pain of TMS.

EQUIVALENTS OF TMS

As has been suggested, other physical disorders may serve the same purpose as TMS. Here is a list of some of the most common ones:

Preulcer states	Tension headache
Peptic ulcer	Migraine headache
Hiatus hernia	Eczema
Spastic colon	Psoriasis
Irritable bowel syndrome	Acne, hives
Hay fever	Dizziness
Asthma	Ringing in the ears
Prostatitis	Frequent urination

All of these disorders should be treated by one's regular physician. Though they may be serving a psychological purpose, they must be investigated and treated medically. Hopefully, the patient will also receive some counseling.

Each of these physical conditions serves equally to assist repression. The more that practitioners identify them as "purely physical," the more they assist in the defense mechanism, which means the continuation of the pain, ulcer, headache, or whatever is going on. As long as the defense works, it will continue.

Physical (as opposed to psychological) defenses against repressed emotions are undoubtedly the most common because they are so successful. They are also very effective, since a patient can transfer from one to another. For example, excellent drugs have been found to reverse the pathology of peptic ulcer. As a result, the mind simply shifts to another physical disorder.

One man in his midforties told me that ten years before, he had started to have trouble with his low back; after many years it was relieved by surgery. A few months after the operation, he began to have stomach ulcer problems, and that went on for almost two years. The doctor tried a number of medications but just couldn't get rid of the ulcer. Finally it stopped, and shortly thereafter, the patient began to have neck and shoulder pain; it had been going on for almost two years and so he had come to see me.

The back surgery and ulcer treatment didn't alleviate his basic problem; they merely acted as placebos and mandated a shift in the location of his physical symptoms.

The Peptic Ulcer Story

The ulcer story is interesting. There has been a decline in the incidence of peptic ulcer in the United States and Canada over the past twenty to thirty years, due in part to the effective drugs that have been developed.

For a better explanation, however, I am indebted to columnist Russell Baker, who asked in one of his Sunday columns in the *New York Times* magazine (August 16, 1981), "Where Have All the Ulcers Gone?" Mr. Baker pointed out that people seemed to be getting fewer ulcers. The article set me to speculating that since everyone, doctors and laymen alike, had come to realize that ulcers really meant tension, they no longer served the purpose of hiding tension, so fewer people developed them. Could this be the reason why neck, shoulder, and back pains have become so common in recent years? Is it possible that these are now much better hiding places for tension than the stomach?

MIND AND BODY

It is my impression that virtually any organ or system in the body can be used by the mind as a defense against repressed emotionality. These include disorders of the immune system, such as hay fever, or frequent respiratory or genitourinary infections. An academic urologist of my acquaintance has said that over 90 percent of his cases of prostatitis are due to tension. I have a patient who suffers from constant dry mouth, the result of tension-induced constriction of his salivary ducts. Laryngitis may be of emotional origin; ophthalmologists tell us that tension-induced visual difficulties are common, and on and on. To repeat, all symptoms should be thoroughly investigated to rule out structural, infectious, or neoplastic processes. This subject is reviewed in more detail in the chapter on mind and body. (See page 155.)

While it is wise to rule out so-called organic disorders, the diagnosis of psychophysiologic conditions should be made positively and not by exclusion. A diagnosis by exclusion is not a diagnosis. It says, "I don't know what this is and therefore it's probably tension induced." Rather the diagnostician should say, "Now that I have eliminated the possibility that there is a tumor or cancer, I can proceed with confidence since this physical condition I am looking at has all the signs and symptoms of an emotionally induced process." That is rarely done, however, for most practicing physicians either do not recognize the disorder as psychophysiologic, or if they do, treat it symptomatically as though it were organic.

The Role of Fear in TMS

Severity of TMS is measured not only by the intensity of the pain but also by the degree of physical disability that exists. What things is the person afraid of or unable to do? Disability may be more important than pain, because it defines the individual's ability to function personally, professionally, socially, and athletically.

In the long run, fear and preoccupation with physical restrictions are more effective as a psychological defense than pain. A severe attack of pain may be over in a few days, but if the person is afraid to do things for fear of inducing another attack or because he or she has found that the activity will invariably bring on pain, even if it is not an acute attack, then the preoccupation with the body is continuous and the defense is working all the time. In the majority of patients with whom I work, this is the most important factor. Occasionally I have a patient who says that he or she has no physical restrictions, that pain is the only problem. But such patients are rare; most patients are afraid of physical activity, which tends to perpetuate the problem by inducing further anxiety and often leads to depression as well. What one sees is truly a *physicophobia*, a fear of physical activity.

The degree of preoccupation with symptoms is a measure of the severity of the problem. Many patients report that the syndrome dominates their lives while others are clearly obsessed by the disorder. It is the first thing they think of when they awaken in the morning and the last at night before sleep comes.

A young woman with whom I was working said one day that she was "terrified of the physical pain." It was clear as we talked, however, that she was really terrified about emotional things, and the pain syndrome had allowed her to avoid them.

It has been my experience that the overall severity of the pain syndrome, including obsessional components, is a good guide to the importance of the underlying emotional state of the patient. By *importance* I mean how much anger and anxiety there are, and how severe the traumas of early life are that have contributed to that person's current psychological state. People who were abused as children, emotionally or physically, but especially sexually, tend to have enormous reservoirs of anxiety and anger. This is one of the first things I think of when I see someone who has a particularly severe TMS. The physical symptoms are the means by which they remain out of contact with some terrible, frightening, deeply buried feelings. Those words are not exaggerations—there is great fear and probably enormous rage festering in their minds that they dare not acknowledge. Such patients will tell you that they understand why the pain will not leave, for when they begin to get close to those buried feelings, they are panic stricken and can proceed no further. They invariably require psychotherapy as part of the therapeutic program.

On the other hand, in the great majority of people with TMS, about 95 percent, the anxiety level and the reasons for it are much milder, and they experience no emotional reaction when the pain disappears. One has the impression in these cases that the mind has overreacted to the anger and anxiety, and the defense wasn't necessary in the first place.

What has been described is universal in our culture; only the degree of repressed emotionality varies. And in our culture, nature has created a mechanism whereby we can avoid being aware of those bad feelings—it gives us physical symptoms.

Fortunately there is a way of stopping what is clearly a maladaptive response for most of us. Logic tells us that the brain is reacting in an infantile fashion. However, my work with TMS has demonstrated that the brain has other attributes and can reverse the process that leads to physical symptoms.

Fear is pervasive. Anything that heightens anxiety will increase the severity of symptoms. One of my patients reported that she left the doctor's office in a state of shock after having been told that the lower end of her spine was degenerating. She said she almost fainted in the street and that her pain was much worse after the visit to the doctor.

A young man in his twenties, with the physique of a football player, told of how he was the strong one in the family business. One day he decided to accompany his father on a visit to a back practitioner since he had experienced some mild low back pain while brushing his teeth. X-rays were taken, and he was told that there was a malalignment of the lower end of the spine, whereupon his mild symptoms got worse. When the pain persisted, he was advised to see a medical specialist, a CT scan (see page 29) was done that showed a herniated disc, and he was now advised that he had a serious problem and that he must do no more heavy lifting, never play basketball again (one of his great loves), and generally be very careful. He was devastated. Though he had started out with mild low back pain, he now had severe pain every day and was greatly limited in his work and life. He had become disabled, thanks to the structural diagnoses that had been made and all that they implied. He now believed there was something seriously wrong with his spine and that he would never again be able to lift a heavy weight or play sports. When I saw him in consultation, he was profoundly depressed.

Fortunately, he had TMS. He responded well to treatment and has been living a normal life again (including playing basketball).

There are many things about having back pain that stimulate fear. The American public is now convinced that the back is a fragile, delicate structure, easily injured and perpetually vulnerable. There are dozens of dos and don'ts: don't bend, don't lift, lift with a straight back, don't sit on a soft chair or couch, don't swim the crawl or breast stroke, don't wear high heels, don't arch your back (which is what the crawl, the breast stroke, and high heels do), sleep on a hard mattress, don't run, no vigorous sports, and so on, ad nauseam. A large group of my successfully treated patients (a few thousand) have demonstrated that these are not valid instructions. All they succeed in doing is to help perpetuate the pain syndrome and make life hell.

There is fear of recurrent attacks. Anyone who has had a severe back attack cannot help but live in terror of the next one. Ironically, by contributing to a high level of anxiety, this fear almost guarantees that another attack will come sooner or later.

Anxiety and anger are enhanced by the perception that you are an inadequate parent, spouse, sexual partner, worker, homemaker, or whatever else you do in life. You can't go to the movies, theater, concert, or restaurant because you can't sit for long. Your woe is double if you are self-employed.

The sad reality is that the patient with back pain is a prisoner of pervasive fear—and fear is a prime perpetuator of the pain syndrome.

Coping

I have heard it said that people get stress-induced pain because they can't cope. It is quite the opposite; TMS occurs because they cope too well. Coping requires that we repress emotions that might interfere with whatever we are trying to do, and TMS exists in order to maintain repression of those emotions.

Someone I saw recently, a high-powered businessman, told me that he can never say no to friends and family who ask him to do things for them, because saying no to him means defeat. Saying yes, and going ahead and accomplishing what he was asked to do, is like winning, no matter what it may cost him emotionally. He is a coper par excellence and a prime candidate for TMS. This also illustrates some of the other characteristics of the TMS personality: the need to be loved, admired, respected; the drive to achieve; and the intense competitiveness. We pay a price for coping—we're great on the outside and we suffer on the inside.

Rejecting the Diagnosis

It is an unfortunate fact that most people would reject the diagnosis of TMS if it were presented to them. This is not surprising, for there remains a strong prejudice in our society regarding anything having to do with psychological problems and psychotherapy. It doesn't matter that the overwhelming majority of such "problems" are minor or that millions of people have psychotherapy every year. Emotional difficulties appear to fall into the same category as racial and religious prejudice.

Judging from the politics of running for public office, the events of recent years suggest that society has done better in overcoming its racial and religious phobias than it has with psychology. We elected John Kennedy. But we have learned from the electoral process in recent years that any hint of a psychological history is still the kiss of death for someone running for high public office. Cruel paradox, for the contemporary political scene suggests that many politicians would profit greatly from psychotherapy. Under the circumstances, it is very unlikely that a politician would acknowledge having TMS.

Similarly, most athletes would reject the diagnosis, since psychological syndromes are equated with weakness, and athletes have an image of strength and indomitability to preserve. I know of a few who have been referred to me but have never come.

Of course, the same prejudice is strong in medicine. Doctors prefer to treat physical disorders; they feel insecure when confronted with patients who have emotional symptoms. Their usual response is to prescribe a medication and hope that the patients will feel better. Even the field of psychiatry now has a large segment of practitioners who prefer to treat primarily with drugs. And I know of a number of psychiatrists who rejected the concept of TMS when it was suggested as a possible explanation for their back pain.

On the other hand, people with physical symptoms rarely encounter such prejudices. Medical insurance will pay for the most elaborate diagnostic and therapeutic procedures, but most policies exclude or sharply limit payment for psychotherapy. Thousands of dollars will be given for an organ transplant to preserve life but peanuts assigned for therapy that will improve the quality of life.

Little wonder that the mind develops strategies to avoid the experience and appearance of emotional difficulty. Unconsciously, we would rather have a physical pain than acknowledge any kind of emotional turmoil.

I discussed this with a patient of mine, who made a cogent observation. She said, "If you ask people to ease up on you because you're emotionally overloaded, don't look for a sympathetic response; but tell them you've got pain or some other physical symptom and they immediately become responsive and solicitous." How right she is. It is perfectly acceptable to have a physical problem in our culture, but people tend to shy away from anything that has to do with the emotions. It is one more reason why the mind will choose a physical rather than an emotional manifestation when confronted with unpleasant emotional phenomena.

IS TMS WORLDWIDE?

From time to time, I have been asked if there are people anywhere in the world who don't get TMS. Dr. Kirkaldy-Wallis, a British-trained physician who worked in Kenya for twenty-two years, provided the answer. He reported at a medical meeting in 1988 that back pain was very rare in indigenous Africans but was just as common in Caucasians and Asians as it is in the United States and Canada. He attributed this partly to cultural differences, positing that Africans didn't seem to generate anxiety as we do. Entirely logical.

THERE'S NOTHING NEW

As the details of this disorder were emerging many years ago, I found it hard to believe that no one had ever seen this problem before. A search of the medical literature turned up an article in a 1946 issue of the *New England Journal of Medicine* by a Major Morgan Sargent describing a large population of returning Air Force personnel who had backache. Dr. Sargent, not a psychiatrist, reported that 96 percent of a large group had psychologically induced pain, and then he went on to describe what was clearly TMS. It was a sign of the times that Dr. Sargent's paper was accepted for publication in the journal. It would probably now be rejected as "unscientific." (I shall elaborate on changing attitudes about mind-body interactions in chapter 7.)

THE SOLUTION

It is at this point that the patient will say, "All right, you've convinced me. I understand why I've got this pain. Now how in the world do I change my personality, solve my problems (especially the insoluble ones, like my ninety-year-old mother), stop generating anger and anxiety, and stop repressing my feelings?"

In fact, Mother Nature has been extremely kind in this instance, for the solution doesn't require any of those difficult transformations in the majority of cases. To be sure, a small number of patients will have to be in psychotherapy to recover, but they represent less than 5 percent of the total. The rest will get better simply by *learning* all about TMS and changing their perceptions about their backs. Does it sound simple? It is and it isn't, as the treatment chapter will detail. (See page 83.)

3

The Physiology of TMS

The word *physiology* refers to the way the various systems and organs of the body work. All biological systems are extremely complicated, and the higher the animal on the evolutionary scale, the more complicated the physiology. This is particularly true with TMS, because this disorder is the result of an interaction between the mental-emotional and the physical spheres of human biology. Medical science has learned an enormous amount about the physiology of most biologic systems in the last one hundred years and about the chemistry and physics of the human body, but virtually nothing is known about interactions between the mind and body, which may be of critical importance in understanding states of both health and disease. TMS appears to be a classic example of mind-body interaction, but we do not understand the chemistry, physics, or cell biology of how emotions can stimulate physical reactions—and yet they do. Here is my concept of how it works in TMS.

THE AUTONOMIC NERVOUS SYSTEM

The physiology of TMS begins in the brain. Here repressed emotions like anxiety and anger set in motion a process in which the autonomic nervous system causes a reduction in blood flow to certain muscles, nerves, tendons, or ligaments, resulting in pain and other kinds of dysfunction in these tissues. The autonomic nervous system is a subsystem of the brain that has the responsibility for controlling all of the body's involuntary functions. It determines how fast the heart beats, how much acid is secreted into the stomach for digestive purposes, how rapidly one breathes, and a host of other moment-to-moment physiologic processes that keep our bodies functioning optimally under everyday circumstances or in emergencies. The so-called fight or flight reaction that all animals share, particularly important in lower animals, is directed by the autonomic system. In order to meet the emergency, every organ and system in the body is properly prepared. For some systems it means total cessation of activity so that the body's resources can be mobilized to deal with the danger more effectively. Typically, most of the body's nutritive and excretory activities are shut down, the heart beats more rapidly, and blood is shunted away from less important functions so as to be available in larger quantities for systems that are crucial to escape or fight, like the muscles. The critical importance of the autonomic system of nerves is obvious.

The autonomic system controls the circulation of blood and does it with the most exquisite precision. It can increase or decrease the flow of blood wherever it chooses and usually does so for good reasons, as described above. But what the system does in TMS we have characterized as an abnormal autonomic activity. It has no useful purpose in the usual sense. It is not contributing to normal daily function or preparing the body for fight or flight. However, it is responding to a psychological need. But we consider what happens to be aberrant, because it results in pain and other distressing symptoms.

OXYGEN DEPRIVATION—THE PATHOPHYSIOLOGY OF TMS

We have postulated that in TMS the autonomic system selectively decreases blood flow in certain muscles, nerves, tendons, and ligaments in response to the presence of repressed emotions like anxiety and anger. This state is known as *ischemia*—that is, the tissue involved is getting less than its normal complement of blood. This means that there will be less oxygen available to those tissues than they are accustomed to, and the result will be symptoms—pain, numbness, tingling, and sometimes weakness. These things happen because of the critical importance of oxygen in all physiologic processes. When it is reduced below its normal levels, one can expect a reaction that will signal that fact.

What is difficult to understand is why the autonomic system should react so as to cause pain and other unpleasant symptoms when its normal function is to keep the body operating at an optimal level regardless of what's going on around it. This is clearly highly unusual but suggests that there must be some pressing need for the reaction. As we have suggested earlier, that need is to deflect the person's attention away from those very unpleasant, often painful emotions that the mind is trying to keep repressed. It is as though the mind had decided that a physical pain is preferable to an emotional one. When viewed in this light, the process is not so illogical.

THE CASE FOR OXYGEN DEPRIVATION

How does one know that oxygen deprivation is responsible for the pain? First, many of the body's reactions to tension and anxiety are the result of abnormal autonomic reactions. The best known is peptic ulcer (a common operation years ago was to cut the autonomic nerves to the stomach as treatment for an ulcer), but so are spastic colitis, tension headache, migraine headache, and a host of others. Therefore, it was thought logical that the pathological physiology of TMS might also originate in the autonomic system.

If the autonomics were to be involved in TMS, the best way that they could produce mischief in muscles and nerves would be through the circulatory system. The small blood vessels bringing blood to these tissues (arterioles) need only be constricted a bit, less blood would reach the area, the tissues would be mildly oxygen deprived, and pain would result.

One body of evidence that the physiologic alteration in TMS is oxygen deprivation is clinical. It has long been recognized that heat, introduced into muscle by diathermy or ultrasound machines, will relieve back pain temporarily. So will deep massage and active exercise of the muscles involved. All three of these physical measures are known to increase blood flow through muscle. Increased blood flow means more oxygen, and if that relieves pain, it is logical to assume that oxygen deprivation was responsible for the pain.

There is also laboratory evidence for this concept. In 1973, two German research workers, H. G. Fassbender and K. Wegner, reported finding microscopic changes in the nuclei of biopsied muscles from back pain patients suggesting oxygen deprivation in "Morphologie und Pathogenese des Weichteilrheumatismus," *Z. Rheumaforsch* (Vol. 32, p. 355).

For additional evidence on the critical role of oxygen in TMS, we are indebted to a group of research workers who have demonstrated in their laboratories in recent years that muscle oxygenation is low in patients suffering from a disorder known as *primary fibromyalgia*. Typical of these reports is one published in the *Scandinavian Journal of Rheumatology* in 1986 (Vol. 15, p. 165) by N. Lund, A. Bengtsson, and P. Thorborg titled "Muscle Tissue Oxygen Pressure in Primary Fibromyalgia." Using an elegant new laboratory tool, they were able to measure muscle oxygen content with great accuracy and found that it was low in the painful muscles of patients with fibromyalgia.

What this means for the etiology (cause) of TMS, as I have long maintained, is that fibromyalgia, also known as *fibrositis* and *myofibrositis* (and to some as *myofasciitis* and *myofascial pain*), is synonymous with TMS. I have treated a large number of patients who came with the diagnosis of fibromyalgia; their medical histories and physical examinations were consistent with severe TMS. As proof that the diagnosis was correct, they recovered completely. Therefore, it is reasonable to maintain that the finding of mild oxygen deprivation in the muscles of patients with fibromyalgia supports the hypothesis that the cause of pain in TMS is the same—oxygen debt.

As mentioned earlier, TMS manifests itself in many ways, both qualitatively and quantitatively, and it is clear that what is called fibromyalgia is one of the ways in which TMS occurs. These patients are among those who suffer the most severe conditions, for they tend to have pain in many different muscles and to suffer from insomnia, anxiety, and depression as well as generalized fatigue. All these manifestations are interpreted as evidence of a higher level of repressed emotionality, primarily anger, and therefore more severe symptoms.

Most contemporary medical investigators cannot accept such an explanation, since it violates their basic presumption that the etiologic explanation for physical abnormalities must be in the body itself. They cannot conceive of the idea that something like back pain might originate in the brain. And therein lies a great tragedy for the patient, for as long as this conceptual recalcitrance persists, the patient will continue to be misdiagnosed.

THE CONSEQUENCES OF OXYGEN DEPRIVATION

Muscle

Oxygen-deprived muscles are painful for two reasons that are known and perhaps others that are beyond our ability to comprehend.

Muscle spasm is the first and most dramatic. It is responsible for the excruciating pain that people experience when they are having an acute attack, as described in the first chapter. However, once the attack has passed, the muscle is not in spasm. In the thousands of patients I have examined through the years, I have rarely found the involved muscles to be in spasm.

The second mechanism, suggested by Dr. Holmes and Dr. Wolfe in a paper published in 1952 titled "Life Situations, Emotions and Backache," published in *Psychosomatic Medicine* (Vol. 14, p. 18), was that the chemistry of the muscles was altered in these patients and that they experienced pain because of a buildup of waste chemicals from the metabolism of lactic acid.

It is of great interest that both muscle spasm and this chemical buildup can be observed in long-distance runners, whose muscles suffer from oxygen deprivation. The presence of muscle pain, either felt spontaneously or induced by the pressure of an examiner's hand, means that the muscle is mildly oxygen deprived. It does not mean that the muscle is "tense." It needs to be emphasized that this oxygen deprivation is usually low level and does not, therefore, damage tissue. This is particularly true of muscle.

Trigger Points

The term *trigger points,* which has been around for many years, refers to the pain elicited when pressure is applied over various muscles in the neck, shoulders, back, and buttocks. There is some controversy over what precisely is painful, but most would agree that it is something in the muscle. Rheumatologists, who have taken the lead in studying fibromyalgia (TMS), appear to avoid using the term, probably because of its association with other diagnoses through the years. I neither use it nor avoid it, for I have concluded that these points of tenderness are merely the *central zones of oxygen deprivation.* Further, there is evidence that some of these points of tenderness may persist for life in TMS-susceptible people, like me, though there may be no pain.

In the first chapter, the point was made that most patients with TMS will have tenderness at six key points: the outer aspect of both buttocks, both sides of the small of the back (lumbar area), and the top of both shoulders. These tender points, trigger points, call them what you will, are the hallmark findings in TMS, and they are the ones that tend to persist after the pain is gone. It is an important part of the physiology of TMS to know that the brain has chosen to implicate these muscles in creating the syndrome we know as TMS.

Patients sometimes ask if breathing pure oxygen will relieve the pain. This has been tried and, unfortunately, does not help. If the brain intends to create a state of oxygen deprivation, it will do so regardless of how oxygen-rich the blood is.

Nerve

Nerve tissue is more sensitive and delicate than muscle. It is likely that oxygen debt causes nerve pain because the reduced level of oxygen threatens the integrity of the nerve, as it does not in muscle. In other words, muscle can withstand a lot of oxygen debt before it will be damaged, far beyond that which occurs in TMS. More sensitive nerve tissue, however, is more easily damaged, and in order to warn the brain that something is wrong, pain begins with very mild oxygen deprivation. We postulate, then, that nerve pain in TMS is a warning signal.

Other nerve symptoms are common in TMS. The person may experience feelings of numbness, tingling, pins and needles, burning, pressure, and others less common. These sensations and the pain are felt in that part of the body served by the nerve.

Nerves are like wires connecting the brain with all parts of the body. They transmit messages from the brain designed to cause muscles to activate and move body parts. But they also transmit messages in the opposite direction, bringing information to the brain about what is going on in the body. For example, if you stick yourself with a pin, impulses travel along nerves informing the brain that something painful has happened. If the nerve is irritated or damaged anywhere along the line, pain will be felt in that part of the body from which these information messages would ordinarily originate. So, for example, if the sciatic nerve is oxygen deprived as it passes through the buttock muscle, one may feel pain in any part of the leg that is served by the sciatic nerve. Since it serves almost the entire leg (one for each leg), there are many varieties of *sciatica*. In some, *sciatica* means pain down the entire back of the leg, in others down the side of the leg. Or the pain may involve only part of the leg or foot, the thigh, the calf, front or back, the top or the bottom of the foot. Sometimes there is pain in the side of the thigh, and then it jumps down to the foot. In occasional cases there is only nerve pain somewhere in the leg or arm, without neck or back pain.

There are patients in whom the upper lumbar spinal nerves are involved, in which case pain may be felt in the upper thigh, groin, or even the lower part of the abdomen. Though the genital organs are served by low sacral spinal nerves, one occasionally sees a patient with scrotal or labial pain whose origin is one of the upper lumbar spinal nerves. A full description of which nerves in the upper or lower back may be involved is to be found in the first chapter.

The nerve fibers that transmit information to the brain are known as *sensory* nerve fibers.

Motor fibers travel in the opposite direction. They bring messages from the brain to the muscles that result in muscle contraction and, therefore, movement. Muscle contraction means that the muscle shortens, which is how it moves a body part. When muscle contracts powerfully and continuously, it is said to be in *spasm,* as described before. It is excruciatingly painful, as it is an abnormal state.

Most nerves, like the sciatic, are mixed nerves. That is, they consist of both sensory and motor fibers. That is why damage to or irritation of a nerve may result in both sensory and motor symptoms, though not necessarily. In

TMS, one sees much variation from patient to patient. There may be only sensory symptoms (pain, tingling, numbness, burning, pressure) or, less common, only motor symptoms (feelings of weakness or real weakness). More often one sees both sensory and motor symptoms.

Tendons and Ligaments

There is much about TMS that is mysterious, and one of the most difficult aspects of the syndrome to understand is the apparent involvement of tendons and ligaments. Tendonitis of the elbow, shoulder, or knee, for example, will often disappear in the course of treatment for TMS. It must be assumed, therefore, that these are part of the syndrome. If that is so, what is the physiologic alteration responsible for the pain?

It has been generally assumed that tendonitis is the result of inflammation, but there is no evidence at all that this is so. Because it is part of TMS, one is tempted to think that oxygen deprivation is at work. Though tendons have no blood vessels, they are living tissue and, therefore, must be supplied with nutrients and oxygen. It is reasonable to assume that the lack of oxygen is also responsible for tendon and ligament pain. Whatever the mechanism, it is clear that these structures are also involved in the charade mounted by the brain in the service of avoiding anxiety and anger, and it is very important to know that tendonitis is one more part of the Tension Myositis Syndrome.

REVIEW

To review the physiology of TMS: It begins with certain emotional states that set in motion activity within the central nervous system, specifically the autonomic system, resulting in local vasoconstriction and mild oxygen deprivation of certain muscles, nerves, tendons, and ligaments. This oxygen lack is responsible for the pain that is the primary manifestation of TMS and the possibility of sensory abnormalities (numbness, pins and needles) and motor deficits such as weakness or tendon reflex changes. (There is much greater detail about which muscles, nerves, tendons, and ligaments are affected in chapter 1.)

Why the mind has chosen to implicate these muscles, nerves, tendons, and ligaments in TMS seems beyond our capacity to comprehend at this time. Indeed, it is likely that at this point in the evolution of the human mind, we are incapable of understanding how the brain works generally, how it comprehends and produces language, how it thinks and remembers, and so forth. Understanding the mechanism of TMS is just one more of the many imponderables of human brain function.

Though it may be of academic interest, knowing the physiology of TMS with certainty is not essential. We know how to stop the disorder, how to "cure" it, for we know its real cause. The chemical and physical changes that take place in the muscles, nerves, tendons, and ligaments that result in pain and other symptoms are the consequences of a process initiated in the brain for psychological reasons. Since any alteration of normal physiology resulting in physical symptoms would serve the same purpose, it is not important to know with precision what is going on in these tissues. As we shall demonstrate in the next chapter on the treatment of TMS, focusing on the physiology and symptomatology of TMS is actually counterproductive, tending to perpetuate rather than alleviate the problem.

4

The Treatment
of TMS

EARLY HISTORY

My treatment of TMS has evolved over the past seventeen years in response to a clear-cut diagnostic concept—that the pain syndromes are the result of the mind-body interaction. When it began to dawn on me that this was the case, my automatic reaction was to explain to the patient what I thought was going on. At the same time, I prescribed physical therapy for everybody, as I had always done. My reasoning was that such therapy could not hurt, and, since I believed that oxygen deprivation was responsible for the symptoms, it might actually be beneficial since all the modalities I prescribed tended to increase the local circulation of blood.

As time went on, something interesting emerged. I found that most of the patients who got better were those who accepted the idea that their pain was the result of emotional factors. Some who improved remained skeptical of the diagnosis but responded well to the physical therapy. It was also apparent that some physical therapists were more successful than others. Based on these observations, two therapeutic conclusions were reached:

1. The most important factor in recovery is that the person must be made aware of what is going on; in other words, that the information provided is the "penicillin" for this disorder.
2. Some patients will respond to physical therapy and/or the physical therapist with a placebo reaction. As has been said earlier, a placebo reaction is fine, but it is usually temporary. Our goal was to effect a complete and permanent cure.

The effectiveness of the placebo reaction was easy to understand, but I was mystified by the obvious importance of informing the patient of what was going on. This was knowledge therapy, and it appeared to make no sense at all. However, I was delighted with its effectiveness, and my cure rate was distinctly better. In addition, I finally had the feeling that I knew what was going on despite my inability to explain all the details. That wasn't too upsetting, for, after all, we were dealing with a process of the brain, and it is common knowledge that little is known about how the brain works.

During this period, I worked closely with a group of talented physical therapists who had learned all about the Tension Myositis Syndrome and combined their physical treatment with discussion of the psychological factors involved. They functioned as surrogates for me as well as physical therapists. It was a painful decision to stop using physical therapy later on, because I so appreciated the work of these dedicated professionals.

Also during those early years, I developed a close working relationship with a small group of psychologists on the staff of the Howard A. Rusk Institute of Rehabilitation Medicine, an association that has continued to this day. I learned a lot of psychology from them, and they have played an important role in the treatment of those patients who needed psychotherapy in order to get better. In essence, we function as a team.

In 1979, perhaps later than I should have, I began to bring groups of patients together for what one might call lecture-discussions. With each passing year, it became increasingly obvious that educating the patient about TMS was the crucial therapeutic factor. Occasionally, I would see a patient who had been psychoanalyzed or had been in psychotherapy for a long time but had a pain syndrome nevertheless. So it was clear that psychological insight was not sufficient to prevent TMS. It wasn't until patients learned the facts about TMS that the pain went away. Starting with four one-hour lectures, we evolved to two two-hour sessions, the first of which is devoted to the physiology and diagnosis of TMS and the second to the psychology of TMS and its treatment. The reason for the lectures was clear—if the information was so important to patients' recovery, then they had to be well educated about TMS. More specifically, it was essential that patients knew exactly what they didn't have (all the structural diagnoses) and what they did have (TMS). From a strictly physical point of view, TMS is harmless; therefore, they had nothing to worry about physically. All the prohibitions and admonitions were unnecessary. Indeed, they actually contributed to the problem by creating fear where none was appropriate.

CURRENT THERAPEUTIC CONCEPTS

If the purpose of the pain is to make one focus on the body, and through these lectures the patient can be convinced to ignore the bodily symptoms and think about psychological things instead, haven't we made the pain syndrome useless?

It's a bit like blowing the cover on a covert operation. As long as the person remains unaware that the pain is serving as a distraction, it will continue to do so, undisturbed. But the moment the realization sinks in (and it must sink in, for mere intellectual appreciation of the process is not enough), then the deception doesn't work anymore; pain stops, for there is no further need for the pain. And it's the information that gets the job done.

The illustration on page 88 should make the point clear. It is in the brain, the organ of the mind, where the unacceptable emotions described in the psychology chapter are generated, hence the arrow up to the right. Straight above, the conscious mind, or what might be called the "mind's eye," is represented. It is in order to prevent the conscious mind from becoming aware of the unpleasant emotions that they are repressed—that is, kept in the unconscious. It must be that something in the mind is fearful that they will not remain repressed, that they are trying to come to consciousness, for it is decided that a *defense* mechanism is necessary, and, psychologically speaking, a defense is anything that will distract the conscious mind (the "mind's eye") from what is being repressed. So the brain creates TMS—the arrow to the left. Now the person must pay attention to all the various manifestations of

86

TMS and can avoid the unpleasantness of experiencing those bad feelings on the right.

This illustration is particularly useful in understanding why one gets rid of TMS by learning about it. If I can convince the conscious mind that TMS is not serious and not worthy of its attention, better yet that it is a phony, a charade, and that rather than fear it one should ridicule it, that most of the structural diagnoses are not valid and that the only things worthy of one's attention are the repressed feelings, what has been accomplished? We will have made the TMS useless; it will no longer have the ability to attract the attention of the conscious mind; the defense is a failure (the cover is blown, the camouflage is removed), which means the pain ceases.

If that all sounds like something out of science fiction or Grimm's fairy tales, one can only say that it works and has worked in a few thousand people over the last seventeen years.

Here's a striking story to illustrate the point. A woman from out of town went through the program and had a good result. Within a few weeks after the lectures, her pain was gone and she resumed all her old activities, including tennis and running. One day about nine months after completing the program, she was out running and developed a pain in a new location, the outer aspect of one of her hips, another manifestation of TMS. Later, she told me the details of the episode.

She saw her local doctor, who said she had bursitis in the hip and put her through X-rays, injections, and medication. She admitted that she was in a lot of pain—and had been for three weeks—while talking on the phone and that I was right to scold her for following her doc-

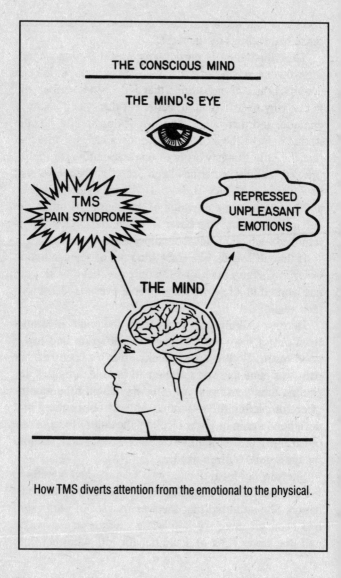

How TMS diverts attention from the emotional to the physical.

tor's regimen. After talking to me, she said she stood for several minutes reflecting, and she got mad—really angry at herself and especially her brain for having pulled that stunt—and she ended up having quite a talk with her brain. Within two minutes, the pain was totally gone and had not recurred. Amazed at how quickly her pain disappeared, she began to jog again, concentrating on the real problem, unconscious anxiety about hurting herself during exercise.

The point of this story is that the information was the crucial factor and that it worked so quickly because she had already been through our program and had integrated (meaning she had accepted at a deeper level) the concepts of TMS. The pain would not have disappeared instantly if she had not already known about TMS. But because she did know about it, because she had been through the lecture program, the moment she realized that the hip pain was another manifestation of TMS, it disappeared because it could no longer successfully hold her attention as a legitimate physical disorder and could no longer distract her from the world of her emotions.

But then you might ask, "Why did she have a recurrence of pain at all?"

The occurrence of pain in TMS always signifies the presence of repressed bad feelings, like anger and anxiety.

"But your program is supposed to prevent this sort of thing from happening; what happened here?"

The fact that this lady developed pain in a new place tells us that her brain was still trying to use the TMS to hide repressed feelings. I discussed this with her, and we agreed that if it happened again, it might be wise to consider psychotherapy. (See page 101 for a discussion of who needs psychotherapy and who doesn't.)

Though this subject has already been discussed in the psychology chapter, it would not be amiss to repeat that there are clearly opposing forces in the mind as to what will be the ultimate fate of these repressed emotions. There must be a force (I can't find a better word) that is trying to bring these feelings to consciousness, despite their unpleasant content. If they were subconscious and destined to remain so, there would be no need for a diversionary process like TMS. The existence of TMS suggests that something is trying to bring these bad feelings to light. One might call this *circular reasoning,* except that there is well-documented evidence in the psychology literature that people exhibit a wide variety of behaviors that are designed to allow them to avoid unpleasant or painful emotional experiences. A classic example is the germ phobia. The person is obsessed with germs and washes his hands a hundred times a day. (Some might call this a compulsion neurosis, but it is the fear of germs that produces the hand-washing compulsion.) Illogical behavior like this has long been recognized as a kind of substitute or displacement for strong, unconscious feelings that the person cannot deal with, hence the preoccupation with germs.

TMS serves the same purpose by keeping one's attention focused on the body, as do a variety of other physical disorders like tension headache, migraine, hay fever, eczema, and heart palpitation, to name a few.

TREATMENT STRATEGIES

The treatment program rests on two pillars:

1. The acquisition of knowledge, of insight into the nature of the disorder.
2. The ability to *act* on that knowledge and thereby change the brain's behavior.

Think Psychological

So one must learn all about TMS, what actually causes the pain, and what part of the brain is responsible—all the things covered in the physiology and manifestation chapters. Then one reviews the psychology of the disorder, the fact that we all tend to generate anger and anxiety in this culture, and that the more compulsive and perfectionistic of us generate a lot. What one must then do is develop the habit of "thinking psychological" instead of physical. In other words, I suggest to patients that when they find themselves being aware of the pain, they must consciously and forcefully shift their attention to something psychological, like something they are worried about, a chronic family or financial problem, a recurrent source of irritation, anything in the psychological realm, for that sends a message to the brain that they're no longer deceived by the pain. When that message reaches the depths of the mind, the subconscious, the pain ceases.

That brings up an important point. Of course, everyone wants the pain to go away immediately. Patients often say,

"All right, I understand very clearly what you're saying—why doesn't the pain stop?"

The last lines of a poem by Edna St. Vincent Millay illustrate the reason why the pain doesn't disappear quickly:

> *Pity me that the heart is slow to learn*
> *What the swift mind beholds at every turn.*

If we substitute the words "subconscious mind" for "heart," the point will be clear. The conscious mind is swift; it can grasp and accept things quickly. The subconscious is slow, deliberate, not quick to accept new ideas and change, which is no doubt a very good thing. Were it not so, humans would be very unstable animals. However, at times like these, when we want things to change quickly, we are impatient with the lumbering subconscious.

Well, how long does it take for the pain to go? Though I am reluctant to talk about numbers, experience has shown that the majority will have resolution of most of their symptoms in two to six weeks after the lectures. Patients are warned, however, that the time may be prolonged if they count the days or weeks or become discouraged if the pain isn't gone when they think it should be gone. Human beings are not machines, and there are many factors tending to vary the time of resolution. How strong are the repressed emotions? How much fear has the person built up over the years? How readily can he or she repudiate the structural diagnoses with which they came?

Talk to Your Brain

Another useful strategy sounds silly at first but has great merit. Patients are encouraged to talk to their brains. So many patients reported having done this on their own with good results that I now routinely suggest it, despite lingering feelings of foolishness. What one is doing is consciously taking charge instead of feeling the helpless, intimidated victim, which is so common in people with this syndrome. The person is asserting himself, telling the brain that he is not going to put up with this state of affairs—and it works. Patients report that they can actually abort an episode of pain by doing this. The woman whose case was described on pages 87–90 did just that and experienced an immediate cessation of pain. It's a very useful strategy.

Resume Physical Activity

Perhaps the most important (but most difficult) thing that patients must do is to resume all physical activity, including the most vigorous. This means overcoming the fear of bending, lifting, jogging, playing tennis or any other sport, and a hundred other common physical things. It means unlearning all the nonsense about the correct way you are supposed to bend, lift, sit, stand, lie in bed, which swimming strokes are good and bad, what kind of chair or mattress you must use, shoes or corset or brace you must wear, and many other bits of medical mythology.

The various health disciplines interested in the back

have succeeded in creating an army of the partially disabled in this country with their medieval concepts of structural damage and injury as the basis of back pain. Though it is often difficult, every patient has to work through his or her fear and return to full normal physical activity. One must do this not simply for the sake of becoming a normal human being again (though that is a good enough reason physically and psychologically by itself) but to liberate oneself from the fear of physical activity, which is often more effective than pain in keeping one's mind focused on the body. That is the purpose of TMS, to keep the mind from attending to emotional things. As Snoopy, that great contemporary philosopher, once said, "There's nothing like a little physical pain to keep your mind off your emotional problems." Charles M. Schulz, the creator of *Peanuts,* is clearly a perceptive man.

I now believe that the physical restrictions imposed by TMS are much more important than the pain, thus making it imperative that the patient gradually overcome them. If patients cannot do this, they are doomed to have recurrences of pain. A few pages back, phobias were mentioned. The pervasive, universal fear of physical activity in people with these pain syndromes, especially of the low back, has prompted me to suggest a new word—*physicophobia*. It is a powerful factor in perpetuating low back pain syndromes.

It should be noted, parenthetically, that the advice to resume normal physical activity, including the most vigorous, has been given to a very large number of patients over the past seventeen years. I cannot recall one person who has subsequently said that this advice caused him or her to have further back trouble.

I suggest to patients that they begin the process of re-suming physical activity when they experience a signifi-cant reduction in pain and when they are feeling confident about the diagnosis. To start prematurely only means that they will probably induce pain, frighten themselves, and retard the recovery process. Patients are usually condi-tioned to expect pain with physical activity and so must not challenge the established programmed patterns until they have developed a fair degree of confidence in the diagnosis.

One of my patients, an attorney in his midthirties, had an interesting experience in this regard. He went through the program uneventfully and in a few weeks was free of pain and doing everything—except one thing. He was afraid to run. He explained to me later that it had been drummed into his head for so many years that running was bad for your back that he simply couldn't get up the courage to try, though he could do many things more strenuous than running. After almost a year, he decided that this was silly and he was going to run. He did, and his pain returned. Now he was at a crossroad; should he continue to run or back off? He called for my advice, but unfortunately I was on vacation, and he had to make his own decision. Wisely, he decided to bull it through. He continued to run and he continued to hurt. Then one night he was awakened from sleep with a very sharp pain in the upper back, but his low back pain was gone. Knowing that TMS often moves to different places during the process of recovery, he decided that he had probably won, and he had. Within a couple of days, the upper back pain was gone, too, and he has not had a recurrence of either upper or lower back pain since that time.

One has to confront TMS, fight it, or the symptoms will continue. Losing one's fear and resuming normal physical activity is possibly the most important part of the therapeutic process.

Discontinue All Physical Treatment

Another essential for full recovery is that all forms of physical treatment or therapy must be abandoned. It is instructive to consider that I did not stop prescribing physical therapy until twelve or thirteen years after I began to make the diagnosis. It took that long for me to fully break with all the old traditions in which I had been schooled. Conceptually, prescribing physical therapy contradicts what we have found to be the only rational way to treat the problem; that is, by teaching, and thereby invalidating, the process where it begins—in the mind. Further, it had become obvious that some patients had put all their confidence in the physical therapy (or therapist) and were having placebo cures (see page 143), which meant that sooner or later, they would be in pain again. The principle is that one must renounce any structural explanation either for the pain or its cure, or the symptoms will continue. Manipulation, heat, massage, exercise, and acupuncture all presuppose a physical disorder that can be treated by some physical means. Unless that whole concept is repudiated, the pain and other symptoms continue.

Patients are usually shocked when it is suggested that they stop the exercises and stretching they have been taught to do for their backs. But it is essential in order to establish firmly in the mind what is important. Exercise for the sake of good health is of course something else, and it is strongly encouraged.

Review the Daily Reminders

This is an important strategy, but one must be careful that it does not become a ritual. Patients are given a list of twelve key thoughts, and it is suggested that at least once a day they set aside fifteen minutes or so when they can relax and quietly review them. They are called daily reminders.

- The pain is due to TMS, not to a structural abnormality.
- The direct reason for the pain is mild oxygen deprivation.
- TMS is a harmless condition, caused by my repressed emotions.
- The principal emotion is my repressed anger.
- TMS exists only to distract my attention from the emotions.
- Since my back is basically normal, there is nothing to fear.
- Therefore, physical activity is not dangerous.
- And I must resume all normal physical activity.
- I will not be concerned or intimidated by the pain.
- I will shift my attention from the pain to emotional issues.
- I intend to be in control—not my subconscious mind.
- I must think psychological at all times, not physical.

By the end of the second lecture-discussion, it is assumed that the information about TMS has been intellectually processed. Patients are then urged to give this information an opportunity to "sink in," to be integrated, to be accepted at a subconscious level, for conscious acceptance, though essential as a first step, is not sufficient to reverse the TMS. Patients are instructed to give it two to four weeks and then call me if they have not made sufficient progress. If they have not, I arrange either to see them in my office or, more commonly, attend a small group meeting composed of patients like themselves (who have made little or no progress) or those having recurrences after having been free of pain for months or years. It is the purpose of these sessions to uncover the reason for the recurrence or lack of progress.

SMALL GROUP FOLLOW-UP MEETINGS

The first thing to ascertain is that the patient understands and accepts the diagnosis. Let's take a theoretical patient, a fifty-year-old businessman. He comes to the meeting because he hasn't improved after attending the lectures. Some of the possible reasons are:

1. He accepts 90 percent of the diagnosis but still has some concerns that the herniated disc demonstrated on the CT scan or MRI has something to do with the pain.
2. He finds it hard to believe that this thing can go away with just an education program.

3. He accepts the diagnosis but can't get up the courage to
begin physical activity.

Mental impediments such as these allow the brain to
continue the TMS, since the man is still engaged with
his symptoms as a physical disorder. As long as he is
in any way preoccupied with what his body is doing,
the pain will continue. His confidence in the diagnosis
needs to be built up so that he can accept the fact that
he has TMS.

The person sitting next to him is a thirty-year-old
homemaker, wife, and mother. She tells us she is no better since the lectures, but she is not surprised because her
life remains as hectic as ever, she is perpetually tired and
harassed, and she never feels as though she has done as
well as she should.

It is pointed out to her that she will never cease being
a perfectionist, that she will always have too much to do,
but that the secret of getting over TMS is not changing
oneself but simply recognizing that the combination of
the realities of her life and personality causes her to generate an enormous amount of anxiety and anger.

Yes, anger too. She has probably never acknowledged
the fact that although she adores her three little girls, she
is simultaneously angry at them for what they require of
her. The idea that she could be subconsciously angry at
her children is outside of her experience. When she grasps
the idea that the cure is in the acknowledgment of such
unacceptable subconscious feelings, the pain will cease.

The man in the back row who next raises his hand
is a forty-five-year-old construction foreman who came
through the program three years ago and had been doing

fine until last week—no pain, no physical restrictions, no problems. Then, out of the blue, he developed an acute low back spasm and now is having severe pain. If he hadn't been through the program, he would really be scared. But he can't understand why this happened.

"What's going on in your life?" I ask him. "Nothing in particular," he says. "My wife is fine, the children are doing well, we don't have any health or financial problems." But the occurrence of an acute spasm means that there has to be something psychological going on, because TMS is an emotional barometer. So I continue to question him, and finally it comes out there have been problems on the job, difficulties with some of the men he supervises, and criticism from his superior.

"Nothing I can't handle," he says, but he doesn't realize that though he's "handling" it, he's generating large quantities of anxiety and anger in the process. There is always important emotional activity going on below the level of consciousness, and we have no way of knowing about it, unless from experience we learn to suspect it and anticipate it.

He leaves the meeting a little wiser about how his emotional insides work. The back pain will subside, and hopefully he will think about his inner reactions the next time he is confronted with a stressful situation.

The small group meetings have proven to be a valuable therapeutic tool. Patients not only gain understanding about their own situations but also profit from the experiences of others. It's always reassuring to know that there are others going through the same thing you are. These meetings also give me an opportunity to decide which patients may need the assistance of a psychotherapist.

PSYCHOTHERAPY

Although about 95 percent of our patients go through the program without psychotherapy, some will need such help. This means simply that they have higher levels of anxiety, anger, and other repressed feelings and that their brains are not going to give up this convenient strategy of hiding these feelings without a struggle. When someone tells me he is having trouble accepting the diagnosis, I suspect that there is resistance in the subconscious to giving up the TMS.

I recall a patient who reported that when he began to become aware of these long-repressed feelings (through psychotherapy), they were so painful and frightening that he was reluctant to deal with them.

These are not people suffering mental illness; these are people who are leading normal, productive lives but who have subconscious emotional baggage that they have never been aware of. Sometimes things happen in childhood that leave one with a large reservoir of resentment and anger, but the feelings are kept deeply buried because they are too scary or socially unacceptable to be allowed to reach consciousness. As has been said before, this tendency to repress bad feelings is universal; it is something we all do to a greater or lesser extent. It is not neurotic—or we are all neurotic.

But in some, as in a person who was abused as a child, the repressed feelings may be strong, and it is necessary for them to have help in recognizing that those feelings are there and in learning how to deal with them. That is the role of psychotherapy.

Unfortunately, society is still backward about the need for and the place of psychotherapy, and there is a common feeling that anyone who needs psychotherapy is weak or incompetent. To harbor repressed feelings has nothing to do with strength of character or mental competence. And yet we are so unenlightened about this matter in the United States that one is virtually ruled out of seeking public office if he or she has ever been in psychotherapy.

It is my own bias that we would be better governed if everyone running for an elective office were *required* to have some psychotherapy. I suspect we might be spared some of the scandals in high places that occur with distressing regularity in our nation.

Two things are emphasized about the need for psychotherapy in our program: Only about 5 percent of the patients will require it; it is no disgrace to be one of the 5 percent.

I have great admiration for the people who go through our program. They must overcome some not inconsiderable impediments before they can get better. One of these is the skepticism and sometimes ridicule they encounter. Another is the constant admonition, usually from family members, to be careful ("Don't lift that," "Don't bend over," "Be sure to put on your corset"). For this reason, I encourage the full participation of close family members so that they will not undermine the therapeutic process.

One of the biggest problems for patients is developing confidence that they can banish this physical disorder with a learning program. That kind of thing is completely outside of people's medical experience. It is my job to convince them that it can be done.

FOLLOW-UP SURVEYS

An important confidence builder is the fact that most people who have gone through the program have been successful. In 1982, we did a follow-up survey on 177 patients who had been treated between 1978 and 1981. Seventy-six percent were leading normal lives with little or no pain, 8 percent were improved, and 16 percent were unchanged. Some of those patients had not had the benefit of lectures, and in many other ways the program was not as sophisticated as it is now.

In 1987, a similar follow-up study was done, this time on a group of patients who all had CT scan–documented herniated discs and had the TMS program between 1983 and 1986. This time, 88 percent (ninety-six people) were successful, 10 percent were improved, and only 2 percent were unchanged.

Still more recently, the well-known journalist-writer Tony Schwartz, who was successfully treated in 1986, mentioned in an article he wrote for *New York* magazine on Dr. Bernie Siegel that he had referred the program to forty patients for treatment and thirty-nine of them were free of pain. I call this Tony Schwartz's miniseries.

A young colleague, Dr. Michael Sinel, at present assistant director of Outpatient Physical Medicine at Cedars-Sinai Medical Center, Los Angeles, has made the diagnosis and treated about fifty patients. His work is noteworthy because included in his patient population are some who were not necessarily receptive to the idea of a tension-induced disorder, making his job much more difficult. Nevertheless, following the basic concepts enunciated in this book, his preliminary data indicate that 75 percent of the group have had good to excellent pain resolution and better than 90 percent have experienced significant functional improvement.

I have invited my colleagues at medical meetings to observe the program and would welcome a survey conducted by an outside organization. Statistics as impressive as mine are bound to evoke skepticism in the medical community.

There is reason to believe the statistics will remain favorable, since I now interview patients prior to consultation in order to discourage those from coming who would not be receptive to the diagnosis. The reality is that only a small proportion of the back pain population would be open to the diagnosis, and it is a waste of time and effort to try to treat someone who could not accept the TMS diagnosis.

Some critics have said that I get such good results because I only accept patients who believe in my concepts. But I can only work with patients who are reasonably receptive to the idea that their emotions are responsible for their pain. Even so, most of my patients are still skeptical when I first see them. It is my job to convince them of the logic of the diagnosis, because only by acknowledging the role of emotions can we get the brain to stop doing what it is doing. That is not believing—it is learning.

Would a surgeon operate on a patient who was not a good surgical risk? Should I be less selective than a surgeon?

Another common criticism by my peers, since we are talking about critics, is that I go too far in claiming that the majority of pain syndromes of the neck, shoulders, and back are due to TMS. "He may be right in 30 percent to 40 percent of the cases," they say.

If 30 percent to 40 percent of back pain patients have TMS, why, then, do these critics *never* make the diagnosis themselves?

The sad fact is that they cannot because it means repudiating long-held diagnostic biases and acknowledging the role of the emotions in these pain syndromes—something for which they have a "visceral incapacity," to borrow a phrase from Senator Byrd of West Virginia.

These treatment results are the only solid proof of the accuracy of the diagnosis and the efficacy of the therapeutic program. Indeed, many of the people who come know one or more successfully treated patients. But that's not new in medicine. The best referral source is still a successfully treated patient.

It should be emphasized I don't consider someone to have been successfully treated unless he or she is free of significant pain (everybody is entitled to a little bit of pain from time to time) and is able to engage in unrestricted physical activity *without fear.* As said before, the fear of physical activity may be more disabling than the pain for someone with a chronic pain problem. Virtually everyone I have seen has been a prisoner of fear (of hurting himself, of bringing on an attack), and that works even better than the pain to keep the attention focused on the body instead of the emotions. It is our job to liberate them from this pervasive fear.

I find myself searching endlessly for ways of getting the message across. Certain phrases may reach some people but not others—so I use them all:

"We're going to try to stop the body from reacting physically to your emotions."

"We want you to learn to send messages to the subconscious mind."

"Information is the penicillin that cures this disorder."

"The cure is knowledge."

"Until now, your subconscious mind has been in charge; I'm going to teach you how to have your conscious mind take over."

"Get mad at your brain; talk to it; give it hell."

"TMS is a trick your mind is playing on you—don't fall for it."

"TMS is a sideshow designed to distract you from what is going on emotionally."

"The symptoms are an act to mask what's going on in the psyche."

"Most of the structural changes in your spine are natural occurrences."

"The brain doesn't want to face up to the repressed anger, so it is running away from it."

"By laughing at or ignoring the pain, you are teaching the brain to send new messages to the muscles."

"We're going to help you take the Sword of Damo-
cles into your hands instead of having it hang
over your head."

I am particularly grateful to a patient, Ms. Norma
Puziss, who presented me with the following verse at the
completion of her treatment program. It is now a regular
part of the lecture-discussion.

Think psychological, not physical,
An idea that is most quizzical.
No one would have guessed
Emotions deeply repressed
Could produce such tension
Not even to mention
TMS.
There is nothing to fear!
Subconscious, do you hear?
You concentrate on pain,
A back sufferer's bane,
To divert one's attention
From underlying tension.
Your secret is out;
You have lost your clout.
So give it up, resign—
TMS is benign!
I am in control, not you.
I have learned that I've got to—
Think psychological, not physical.

I am sure that this wonderful bit of verse has been helpful to many of my patients, since it captures one of the basic ideas so beautifully.

Since it is characteristic of people with TMS to feel victimized and not in control, the treatment program must help them regain their sense of power by pointing out that the source of the pain is a harmless process. I encourage patients to develop an attitude of disdain toward the pain to replace their strong feelings of intimidation. This sends a message to the subconscious that the strategy of keeping attention focused on the body is about to fail—which means the cessation of pain.

QUESTIONS PEOPLE ASK

One of the more difficult concepts to grasp is the fact that one does not have to eliminate tension from one's life.

People ask, "How do I change my personality, and how do I stop generating anxiety and anger?"

If these were prerequisites for recovery, my cure rate would be zero. It is not changing one's emotions; it is recognizing that they exist and that the brain is trying to keep one from being aware of their existence through the mechanism of the pain syndrome. That is the key point in understanding why the knowledge is the effective cure.

"How do you know that what you're doing is not a placebo?"

An excellent question and one that has always concerned me, because a placebo reaction is to be assiduously avoided. A placebo cure is almost always temporary, and we are looking for permanent resolution of the pain. Therefore, we would not be satisfied with a placebo cure. This is all too common. People are administered a large variety of physical treatments, feel better for a few days, and then need another treatment. (And, of course, they never overcome their fear of physical activity.) One of the reasons I know the TMS program does not induce a placebo reaction is the fact that almost all patients have permanent resolution of symptoms.

A second reason is that the placebo effect is based on blind faith; patients know little or nothing about the disorder they have and the rationale for treatment. They simply trust the treating practitioner. The educational program employed in the treatment of TMS is the very opposite. I teach patients literally all I know about the disorder; they are encouraged to ask questions, and they are warned that they must find the diagnosis logical and consistent. Their recovery depends on information, on awareness. They are active participants in the recovery process. This is anything but a placebo process.

Perhaps the most compelling argument that what we do is not a placebo is the fact that on numerous occasions since the publication of the book *Mind Over Back Pain,* the predecessor of this one, people have reported complete and permanent resolution of pain simply by reading the book. There is no personality influence here, no bedside manner; just plain, solid information. And we have learned that that's what it takes to banish TMS.

"Why have you stopped using physical therapy as part of your treatment program?"

This was touched on before but it bears repeating. As has just been said, any physical treatment can be a placebo, including physical therapy, and we strive to avoid this because the result is temporary. But there is another, more subtle reason. If I am trying to get people to stop paying attention to their bodies and start thinking psychologically about their pain, am I not contradicting my own therapeutic strategy if I prescribe physical therapy? It took me a long time to realize this and get up the courage to stop prescribing it, for, after all, I was taught to depend on physical treatments like everyone else. I only remember with some effort now how difficult it was to start "going pure"—that is, to depend on the education program exclusively. In fact, to emphasize the point, I recommend to patients that they stop doing all exercises that are designed to protect or help the back, for the same reason. They must do *nothing* to focus attention on the painful area.

In this same vein, patients are taught that there is no correct way to bend or lift, one doesn't need to avoid soft chairs or mattresses, corsets and collars are unnecessary, and in general the great number of admonitions and prohibitions that have become part of back pain folklore are simply without foundation, because TMS is a harmless condition, and there is nothing structurally wrong with the back. Running is not bad for the spine; weak abdominal muscles do not cause back pain; strong back muscles do not prevent back pain; it is perfectly all right to arch the back, swim the crawl or breast stroke; man *was* meant to walk upright (*Homo sapiens* and his ancestors have

110

been doing so for somewhere between 3 and 4 million years); a short leg does not cause back pain. One could go on and on.

"How can I tell the difference between TMS and pain from overworking unused muscles?"

That's easy. When you've done some unaccustomed physical activity and wake up the next morning with aches in your arms or legs, it's a good kind of ache and it's usually gone by the following day. The pain of TMS is always nasty, and it doesn't go away very quickly, if at all.

"What kind of exercise can I do?"

When the pain has subsided, one can do anything and everything, the more strenuous the better. Obviously one should follow a strenuous routine only after consulting with one's doctor. But the point is that exercise should be done for general health reasons, not for the back.

"Suppose the pain goes away in my low back and starts up in the neck and shoulders. What do I do?"

My routine advice to patients is to call me up so that we can discuss the meaning of the switch. During the early phases of the treatment program, the brain may try to locate the TMS somewhere else in the neck, shoulders, back, or buttocks. It is reluctant to give up this convenient strategy for diverting attention away from the emotions. Patients must be warned that this may occur, that they must not panic or get discouraged but merely apply the same principles to the new location. I remind them that the musculoskeletal system is not the only one where the brain can set up a diversion. It can do the same thing in the gastrointestinal tract; the head, with tension or migraine headache; the skin; the genitourinary tract. The brain can cause mischief in any organ or system in the body, so one must be on guard. I advise my patients to consult their regular physicians if a new symptom occurs but to let me know about it since it may be serving the same purpose as TMS. For example, stomach ulcers should be treated with proper medication, but it is almost more important to recognize that they are coming from tension factors.

"What do I do if I get a recurrence six months or a year from now?"

I advise patients to call me immediately so that we can promptly start looking for the psychological reason for it. This usually means attendance at one of the small group meetings or a visit to my office.

"What about hypnosis? Isn't that a good way to get your mind to do what you want it to do?"

On a temporary basis, yes, but we are looking for a permanent cure. Just recently, a study done at Stanford Medical School and reported in the *American Journal of Psychiatry* demonstrated very nicely that with hypnosis, pain could be markedly diminished in some patients. That is desirable if you are treating pain, as in patients with cancer. But I tell my patients, with considerable agitation, that *I don't treat pain!* That would be symptomatic treatment, and it's poor medicine. I treat the disorder that is the root cause of the pain. To the best of my knowledge, hypnosis would not contribute to that process.

Which leads to a subject I would rather not discuss, it pains me so. But discuss it we must, for it is of great importance. It has to do with how "chronic pain" is treated in the hundreds of pain clinics established in the last twenty years across the country.

The basic principle, first enunciated by a nonphysician, is that chronic pain is a separate disease entity, an exaggeration of the pain of some persistent structural abnormality that develops because patients derive what psychologists call "secondary gain" from the pain. That is, the pain brings them some psychological benefit, like attention, money, or escape from the world. It is theorized that patients learn this behavior because it is encouraged by the medical system, family, and friends. Treatment is designed to discourage this by rewarding nonpain behavior and "punishing" its opposite. Students of psychology will recognize these ideas as deriving from the work of B. F. Skinner, who became widely known for his work in demonstrating this kind of conditioning.

While it is well known that human beings can be conditioned in the classic Pavlovian sense, one must be very careful about applying Skinnerian principles to human beings. Elements of secondary gain are often identified in my patients, but they are by no means the primary psychological factors at work. To attribute to secondary gain such importance is to ignore the real problem—repressed feelings of all kinds—and make the equally egregious mistake of failing to recognize the true physiology of the pain, that it is not due to a persistent structural abnormality but to a psychophysiologic process, as described in this book.

It is for this reason that these pain clinics sometimes help but rarely cure their patients.

"Is the TMS treatment program an example of vis medicatrix naturae, *or the body's ability to heal itself?"*

In one sense it certainly is. But in another, it goes beyond the usual process of self-healing that is always at work when we are injured or invaded by poisons or infectious agents. This is an example of how a particular kind of physical disorder, a psychophysiological process, can be reversed. In the last chapter, we shall discuss this and other mind-body interactions, a subject that is finally beginning to command the attention of research medicine.

5

The Traditional (Conventional) Diagnoses

Though I find the chore distasteful, it is essential to review the large number of disorders to which neck, shoulder, back, and limb pain are routinely attributed. The reader should know what these diagnoses mean to the people who make them, to the many disciplines that treat them, and to the people who are diagnosed as having them.

In the course of my lectures to patients with TMS, it is made clear that it is important to know what's causing the pain and what is *not* causing it, because many of the diagnoses to be described evoke great fear, and, as the preceding chapters make clear, fear is a dominant factor in worsening and perpetuating the pain syndrome.

The average citizen in this country believes that the low back is a vulnerable, fragile structure, easily injured and constantly prone to reinjury. As that perception widens, the occurrence of back pain in the population increases so that now one repeatedly hears the astonishing figure that 80 percent to 85 percent of adults have a history of one of these pain syndromes. Ideas about the vulnerability of the back are, to a large extent, based on the diagnoses practitioners make. Such words as *herniation, degeneration, deterioration,* and *disintegration,* constantly used to describe the lower end of the spine, provoke fear and provide a ready explanation for the "injury" and the attack of excruciating pain. Further, there are dozens of prohibitions and admonitions people learn in their interaction with physicians and other practitioners, and sometimes from family and friends, like these:

Don't bend.
Don't slouch.
Don't sit on soft chairs or couches.
Don't arch your back.
Don't swim the crawl or breast stroke.
Don't wear high heels.
Always lift with a straight back.
Running is bad for your spine.
Never run on hard surfaces.
Weak back muscles cause back pain.
Strong abdominal muscles protect you from back pain.
Always stretch before exercising.
If you have back pain, avoid all vigorous sports.

This is only a partial list. Because of a basic misconception of the cause of neck, shoulder, and back pain, there is a monumental body of misinformation to which people are exposed and that contributes substantially to the severity and longevity of their painful episodes.

The truth is that the back is a rugged structure, fully capable of taking us through our daily lives, and then some. We exercise our backs constantly, for the act of being up and about requires that the *postural muscles,* which paradoxically are the only ones involved in TMS, are always active in keeping the trunk upright on the legs and the head on the trunk. And if we take a brisk walk, or jog, or run, those muscles are exercised even more. They are undoubtedly the strongest muscles in the body.

When I hear that a professional athlete, a tennis player, for example, has had to pull out of a tournament because of back pain, I marvel at the naïveté that suggests that he or she has a deficient back. Such a thing was practically unheard of thirty years ago in tennis, golf, baseball, football, or basketball. It is commonplace today.

Years ago, I saw a famous woman athlete who was having pain in the very muscles she used most in her sport. Fortunately, she immediately grasped the concept of TMS, and her pain promptly disappeared.

COMMON STRUCTURAL DIAGNOSES

In my experience, structural abnormalities of the spine rarely cause back pain. That ought not surprise us, for this epidemic of back pain is very new. Somehow the human race managed to get through the first million years or so of its evolution without a problem, but if the structural diagnoses are correct, something happened to the spine during the last evolutionary eyeblink, and it has begun to fall apart.

This idea is untenable. One suspects that these spine abnormalities have always been there but were never blamed for pain, because there was no pain to blame them for. Fifty years ago, back pain was not very common, but, more importantly, nobody took it seriously. The epidemic of back pain is due to the enormous increase in the incidence of TMS during the past thirty years, and, ironically, the failure of medicine to recognize and diagnose it has been a major factor in that increase. Instead of TMS, the pain has been attributed primarily to a variety of structural defects of the spine.

It's essential to know that almost all of the structural abnormalities of the spine are harmless. With that in mind, let's take a look at the common conventional diagnoses.

Herniated Disc

Though the back sufferer isn't aware of it, it is generally known by students of the spine that the last intervertebral disc, between the fifth lumbar vertebra and the sacrum, is more or less degenerated in most people by the age of *twenty*. Discs are structures located between the bodies of spinal bones to take up the shock. They are firmly attached to the vertebral bodies above and below, and in no way can they "slip." Enclosed by a tough, fibrous outer shell, there is a thick fluid inside, which is what absorbs the shock. The discs at the lower end of the spine and in the neck, because of all the activity in those locations, begin to wear out at an early age, some by the age of twenty, as stated.

Although no one knows exactly what happens, the disc gets flatter, suggesting that the fluid inside has dried up or broken through a weakened part of the disc wall, usually toward the back. This breaking through the disc wall is what is known as a *disc rupture* or, more commonly, *herniation*. It is probably similar to squeezing toothpaste from a tube. In some cases, the fluid does not break through but merely bulges the wall. All of these things can be seen on a CT scan or MRI, remarkable diagnostic techniques that show soft tissue detail. Conventional X-rays only show bone unless a contrast material is used.

The important question is, "What harm is done by this extruded disc material, if any?"

The conventional idea is that the "toothpaste" compresses a nearby spinal nerve, thereby producing pain. If it is the disc between lumbar vertebrae 4 (L4) and L5, or L5 and the sacrum, the pain will be in the leg. If in the neck, there is arm pain. The leg pain is usually called *sciatica*.

It has been my experience that herniated disc material is rarely responsible for pain or any other neurological symptom. This is a minority opinion, but I am not totally alone. A well-known neurosurgeon and chairman of his department at the University of Miami School of Medicine, Dr. Hubert Rosomoff, has come to a similar conclusion, discussed in his article "Do Herniated Discs Produce Pain?," published in *Advances in Pain Research and Therapy* and edited by H. Fields, R. Dubner, F. Cervero, and L. Jones (New York: Raven Press, 1985). He did back surgery for many years and apparently bases his conclusion on observed inconsistencies and the logical fact of neurological pathophysiology that continued compression of a nerve will cause it to stop transmitting pain messages after a short time. The result is numbness. How could the herniation then cause continuing pain?

Another highly respected physician and investigator who studied the problem for years, Dr. Alf Nachemson of Sweden, concluded in his article "The Lumbar Spine: An Orthopedic Challenge," published in 1976 in *Spine* (Vol. 1, p. 59), that the cause of back pain was unknown in the majority of cases, and almost all should be treated nonsurgically.

My conclusion that most disc herniations are harmless is based on seventeen years of treating such patients with a high degree of success, leading to the impression that the extruded material is not hurting anything; it's just there.

The innocence of the poor, maligned disc was first suspected when a frequent lack of correlation was noted between what one would expect the disc herniation to do and what was found on taking a history and doing a physical examination.

For example, the diagnostic study (CT scan or MRI) might show a herniated disc at the interspace L4–L5, one of the possible consequences of which might be weakness in the muscles that elevate the foot and the toes. The examination, however, revealed that not only those muscles were weak but so were the ones in the back of the leg, muscles that are not energized by the spinal nerve passing by interspace L4–L5. Then when I found on examination that the buttock muscles in the vicinity of the sciatic nerve were painful to pressure, it was apparent that the nerve disturbance was not coming from the region of the herniated disc but from the sciatic nerve that serves both sets of muscles. The following case history illustrates this:

The patient was a forty-four-year-old professional woman with a fifteen-year history of recurrent low back and leg pain. About seven months prior to consultation, she had a severe attack with pain in the low back and right leg. She also complained of weakness in the right leg.

A CT scan demonstrated a small herniation of disc material between the fifth lumbar vertebra and the sacrum that must have been extruded a long time ago for it was calcified. It didn't look capable of causing symptoms, but that was the diagnosis. Pain continued during the intervening seven months, and she was restricted physically because of the weakness in the right leg.

My examination disclosed an absent right ankle tendon reflex and weakness of the right calf muscles. Both of these findings could be explained by pressure on the first sacral spinal nerve (which is what the original doctor claimed), since that nerve sends motor fibers to the calf muscle and does pass in the vicinity of the disc in question. However, further examination showed that the muscles on the front of the leg were also weak; she had partial foot drop. This could not be ascribed to the disc herniation, because the spinal nerves supplying these muscles were not near the herniation.

On the other hand, all of the findings could be explained by something interfering with normal function of the right sciatic nerve, as commonly seen with TMS. That nerve receives branches from spinal nerves lumbar 3, lumbar 4, lumbar 5, sacral 1, and sacral 2. Therefore, anything that disturbs the sciatic nerve may affect the parts of the leg supplied by any or all of those nerves, which was clearly the case with this patient.

Her examination also revealed tenderness on pressure

over all the muscles of the right buttock, which is where the sciatic nerve is located. This and other characteristic findings on physical testing established the diagnosis of TMS involving the right buttock and sciatic nerve; the herniated disc was an incidental finding of no significance.

Such clinical discrepancies are common and make one wonder why they are not routinely discovered.

So fixed are physicians on the herniated disc, the diagnosis is sometimes made solely on the basis of a history of simultaneous low back, buttock, and leg pain, or even in the absence of leg pain, without benefit of a CT scan or MRI study. The diagnosis of herniated disc cannot be made clinically or even with plain X-rays. If the latter are done, what is usually seen is narrowing of an intervertebral disc space, most frequently of the last two intervertebral spaces. At the last space, this abnormality is almost universal beyond the age of twenty, as stated earlier. It means the disc has degenerated, and it is a perfectly normal part of the aging process. It may be tempting but is inadvisable to attribute symptoms to normal aging phenomena. In my experience, disc degeneration is no more pathological than graying hair or wrinkling skin.

In recent years, there have been numerous reports in the medical literature of herniated discs in patients with no history of back pain. They were discovered inadvertently on CT or MRI studies done to investigate other parts of the body.

In fairness to an objective evaluation of the problem, it should be noted that in one statistical study, there was a higher incidence of back pain historically in people with evidence of disc abnormalities. I have tried to reconcile this with the clear observation that it is TMS and not disc pathology that causes the pain and can only conclude that in the mysterious process by which the brain chooses a site for TMS, it selects an area of "abnormality" (like disc herniation) even though the anatomical aberration may not be pathological.

In order to document the large number of herniated disc patients treated successfully over many years, a follow-up survey was conducted in 1987. One hundred and nine patients were interviewed by telephone by a research assistant. Their names were selected randomly from a large population of patients who were seen and treated from one to three years previously. In each case, pain was attributed to a herniated disc that could be seen on CT scan. Based on history and physical examination, the diagnosis was TMS; all went through the usual treatment program. The results were as follows:

Free, or nearly free of pain, unrestricted
    physical activity .... 96 (88 percent)
Improved, some pain, restricted activity ...... 11 (10 percent)
Unchanged 2   (2 percent)

The two patients who did not improve were found to have severe, persistent psychological problems and continue in psychotherapy to this day.

These statistics make it difficult to take the herniated disc seriously. Yet each of these patients had been told that this was the reason for the pain; thirty-nine had been advised to have surgery; three had already had such surgery; and most of the rest had been told that surgery might be necessary if conservative measures failed.

Here is another case history. The patient was a twenty-year-old man with a history of low back and right leg pain; he had had a lumbar myelogram showing a herniated disc two months before I saw him in consultation. He was advised to stop all physical activity, and surgery was recommended, both appropriate recommendations if the disc was the cause of the pain. A dedicated athlete (basketball and squash were his favorites), he was devastated by the diagnosis. He was further upset by the fact that he would no longer be able to "burn off" his tension through vigorous sports, and he saw himself as a very tense fellow.

He decided against surgery and, with great trepidation, continued to work out in the gymnasium; he even played basketball occasionally. Though he got neither better nor worse, he lived in constant fear that he might really hurt himself.

My examination disclosed no evidence of nerve damage in either leg; the straight leg–raising test on both sides caused pain in the right buttock. As usual with TMS, there was pain on manual pressure over the muscles of both buttocks, the small of the back on both sides, the top of both shoulders, and the sides of the neck. These findings indicated that the pain was due to TMS and not the herniated disc. He accepted the diagnosis, participated in the treatment program, and was free of pain in a few weeks. It is now about twelve years since that patient was seen, and he has continued to do well despite his vigorous physical program.

Spinal Stenosis

During the years that I have been engaged in this work, I have seen the diagnosis of *spinal stenosis* emerge as one of the most common when there is low back pain and no herniated disc to blame. It refers to narrowing of the spinal canal, occasionally thought to be congenital but most often as a result of aging in the spinal bones. Buildup of bone, in some places called *osteophytes,* narrows the canal.

My reaction to this abnormality is based on experience with patients. Most of those I have seen, regardless of age, were found to have TMS, which allowed me to disregard the X-ray diagnosis. When stenosis is severe, the canal should be widened surgically, but I have seen very few of such cases.

It is my practice, particularly with older patients, to suggest neurological consultation so that the possibility of significant impingement on neural structures can be carefully studied. If the neural picture is satisfactory and the patient has the classic findings of TMS, I proceed with confidence regardless of what the X-ray shows.

Pinched Nerve

After herniated disc, a *pinched nerve* is one of the most common diagnoses made, usually when patients present with pain in the neck, shoulder, and upper limb on the same side. What is presumably being pinched is a cervical spinal nerve as it courses its way through a hole formed by contiguous cervical vertebrae (known as a *foramen*), and what is supposed to be doing the pinching is an osteophyte (see above—a buildup of bone, a bone spur) or a herniated disc.

The diagnosis is fraught with difficulty; it rests on exceedingly shaky concepts. Once more, the need to identify a structural cause is the problem and sometimes breeds a disturbing lack of objectivity. The following observations throw doubt on the pinched nerve diagnosis.

First, these symptoms often occur in young adults, who have no bone spurs and no herniated discs.

Second, bone spurs are extremely common, and many people who have them don't have pain. Spurs increase in number and size with advancing age, so that by late middle age and beyond, everyone ought to have neck and arm pain from them, but everyone doesn't.

Third, neuroradiologists (specialists in X-rays of the nervous system) tell us the spurs would have to obliterate the foramen before compression of the nerve would occur, something one rarely sees.

Fourth, the same principle applies here as with the lumbar herniated disc: Persistent compression of a nerve will produce objective numbness (absence of pain on testing). This is different from the subjective sensation of numbness that patients sometimes feel in a leg or arm.

Fifth, there are numerous reports in the medical literature of large growths in the spine, like benign tumors, that often produce no pain.

Most "pinched nerve" patients have TMS involving the muscles of the neck and shoulders, particularly the upper trapezius muscle and the cervical spinal nerves *after they have left the spinal bones*. Four cervical and the first thoracic spinal nerves form what is known as the *brachial plexus,* a kind of staging area, where they are then reorganized into the nerves that go into the arm and hand. It is highly likely that the brachial plexus is often implicated in the TMS process. But whether it is the spinal nerves, the brachial plexus, or both is irrelevant, for we do not treat the disorder locally; we work on it where it begins—in the brain.

Here is a striking case history that teaches many lessons. The patient was a middle-aged professional woman who developed pain in the left neck, shoulder, and entire left arm, with particularly severe pain in the wrist. She was often awakened at night by the wrist pain. To make matters worse, she realized one day that she had lost almost all movement at the left shoulder, what's known as a "frozen shoulder." This is a common complication of shoulder pain. Patients apparently begin to limit movement at the shoulder, probably because of pain, without realizing that they're not moving it, and are suddenly aware that the range of motion is gone. In the absence of normal movement, the capsule of the shoulder joint shrinks, as it will in any joint in which there is restricted movement. Further, she reported that the left hand was weak, and she tended to drop things.

Despite the ominous sound of these symptoms, I suspected she had TMS and the physical examination supported the diagnosis. The patient was receptive to the diagnosis. She was familiar with the syndrome and fit the psychological profile perfectly: she was overcommitted professionally, extremely hardworking, and compulsive about her responsibilities.

To my embarrassment, the symptoms did not respond

to the usual therapeutic program; on the contrary, they continued to be severe for many weeks. Thinking there might be something serious going on that was mimicking TMS, I arranged for a neurologic consultation. The physical examination and all tests were normal.

After many weeks, the symptoms began to subside, and as they did, we both realized why they had started in the first place and why she was now getting better. The trouble began when she was informed that she was going to lose a very important member of her research team. In anticipation of that event, an enormous amount of work had to be done and she dreaded her departure—hence a great deal of anxiety and undoubtedly a lot of deep-down anger at this unfortunate turn of events was generated. The subconscious mind is not particularly logical about such things.

Total disappearance of symptoms coincided with the actual departure of the valued colleague, suggesting that with the fait accompli there was no longer any need for the TMS. She regained full range of motion of the shoulder without benefit of physical therapy.

This was a classic "pinched nerve" diagnosis—except that it wasn't. As the case clearly demonstrates, TMS exists in the service of psychological phenomena. To attribute symptoms to a structural abnormality is a sad diagnostic error.

The Facet Syndrome

Facet is the technical name for a joint between two spinal bones. Like all joints, they are subject to wear and tear and begin to look abnormal as we get along in years. It is believed that these changes cause pain in some patients. In my experience they do not.

Arthritis of the Spine

What is generally meant when the term *arthritis of the spine* is used is *osteoarthritis* or *osteoarthrosis*. These refer to the normal aging changes we have been talking about. They are also referred to as *spondylosis*. I have not found that this is pathological, therefore, not productive of symptoms. Rheumatoid arthritis is an entirely different matter. It is an inflammatory process that can strike at any joint in the body and is always painful.

Transitional Vertebra

Transitional vertebra is a congenital abnormality in which there is an extra bone at the lower end of the spine, usually attached to the pelvic bone. It often gets the blame when found in the presence of back pain.

Spondylolysis

Spondylolysis is another defect in a vertebral bone, easily detected on X-ray and rarely responsible for back pain in my experience.

Spina Bifida Occulta

Spina bifida occulta is still another congenital abnormality at the end of the spine, but in this one there is a piece of bone missing. Once more, pain is historically (but mistakenly) attributed to this defect.

Spondylolisthesis

Spondylolisthesis is an abnormality in which two vertebral bones, usually at the lower end of the spine, are not correctly aligned with each other. One is in front of the other. It is a scary-looking thing on X-ray, but I have found it to be uniformly benign. It is of course possible that there are some that are not benign, but thus far I have not seen one such.

There have been some pretty dramatic cases over the years. I recall a man in his late fifties with a three-year history of increasing back pain that was the bane of his existence, to use an old cliché. He couldn't participate in sports, which he missed badly, and he described his days as "pure torture." Though surgery was recommended more than once, he was afraid of it despite his desperate condition.

The examination revealed an extremely anxious man, though quite healthy-looking. There were no neurological changes in his legs, but all of the muscles from his neck to his buttocks were exquisitely tender to pressure. He was a classic case of TMS.

Here was a dilemma: One patient with two diagnoses,

spondylolisthesis and TMS. I had no doubt that the pain was due to the TMS, and the patient said he wanted to believe me, but what about the doctors who recommended surgery—could they be wrong? I suggested that since he obviously had TMS, we should try to rid him of that pain and see what was left.

The usual course of treatment was begun, and the pain began to diminish. About four weeks into the program, he went on a vacation with his wife and reported on his return that he had been totally free of pain during the entire holiday. Upon his return to New York and the resumption of his usual life, the pain returned but to a milder degree. There was no longer any question about the cause of his pain. He continued to improve and three months after his first visit resumed his favorite sport.

The man wrote me on his first anniversary of having consulted with me and all was still well. He was playing his game competitively and considered his recovery remarkable in view of the fact that his treatment consisted only of listening and learning.

It would be imprecise to say that spondylolisthesis never causes back pain; but, thus far, I have not seen a patient in whom it did.

Between 1976 and 1980, two Israeli physicians, Dr. A. Magora and Dr. A. Schwartz, published four medical articles in the *Scandinavian Journal of Rehabilitation Medicine* in which they reported the results of studies they had done to determine whether certain spinal abnormalities caused back pain. Their method was to compare the X-rays of people with and without a history of back pain. If people with back pain had these abnormalities more commonly, one could presume that the abnormalities might be the cause of the pain.

They found no statistical difference in the incidence of degenerative osteoarthritis, transitional vertebra, spina bifida occulta, and spondylolysis between the two groups. There was a small statistical difference for spondylolisthesis. In other words, one could not attribute back pain to these disorders, with the possible exception of spondylolisthesis.

A similar study was conducted by American radiologist Dr. C. A. Splithoff and published in the *Journal of the American Medical Association* in 1953. He compared the incidence of nine different abnormalities of the end of the spine in people with and without back pain. Again he found no statistical difference.

These studies suggest that structural abnormalities of the spine do not generally cause back pain.

Scoliosis

Scoliosis refers to an abnormal curvature of the spine commonly seen in teenage girls and usually persisting into adult life. Its cause is unknown. It rarely causes pain in teenagers but is often blamed for back pain in adults. I have not yet found this to be the case. The following case history is typical.

The patient was a woman in her thirties who had suffered recurrent attacks of back pain since her teens. Several years before I saw her, she had experienced a severe attack at a time when she was taking care of her young children. Mild scoliosis, to which the pain was attributed, was seen on X-rays. She was told her back pain would gradually worsen as she got older. Despite this dire prediction, she recovered from that episode and did fairly well until two months before I saw her, when she had a bad attack. She said it began when she was bending over and "felt something snap," a common description of onset, as described earlier in the book. She was further frightened because her trunk was tilted to one side.

On taking her history, I learned that over the years she had experienced a number of episodes of tendonitis in the arms and legs, occasional pain in the neck and shoulders, stomach and colon symptoms, hay fever, and severe headaches. A classic TMS patient.

The physical examination was normal except for the usual tenderness on palpation of muscles in the neck, shoulders, back, and buttocks.

She had no trouble accepting the diagnosis, participated in the treatment program, and was soon pain free. She later reported that there had been no more attacks, that she sometimes had mild pain but knew it was harmless and went about her life without fear.

It is clear that scoliosis was not the source of her pain, since nothing in the treatment changed the scoliosis. It is equally clear that her personality predisposed her to a variety of benign physical ailments, including TMS.

Osteoarthritis of the Hip

Osteoarthritis of the hip is well known among laymen because it is common and because of the dramatic surgical procedure in which the entire hip joint is replaced;

the patient gets a new socket and a new ball (the head of the femur) to fit into it. This is certainly one of the great triumphs of reconstructive surgery.

What necessitates this operation is the overgrowth of bone and the wearing away of the cartilage of the joint so that it loses range of movement and becomes dysfunctional. It is also alleged that these osteoarthritic joints are painful, and that may be so in some cases. One must, however, be very careful, for I have seen a number of patients whose "hip" pain was clearly due to a manifestation of TMS.

Just recently I saw such a case. The patient was a woman in her sixties who complained of hip pain. X-ray of the hip joint showed only moderate osteoarthritic change (to which the pain had been, nevertheless, attributed), but the physical examination told the tale. She had perfectly normal range of motion in the joint, and there was no pain with weight bearing on that leg. The site of the pain was located about two inches above the joint and could be reproduced by direct pressure. What she had was tendonalgia due to TMS.

Frequently the pain will come from buttock muscle or the sciatic nerve involved with TMS. I can say this with some confidence, because I treat these people and their pain goes away. I do not say that this is invariable but merely that one must be alert to the possibility that hip pain is not always due to a degenerated hip joint.

Chondromalacia

Chondromalacia is a roughening of the underside of the patella (kneecap), demonstrable on X-ray, which is no doubt the reason why it is routinely blamed for knee pain. Unlike what has just been said about hip osteoarthritis, this is a disorder that never, in my experience, causes pain. Invariably the examination discloses evidence of TMS tendonalgia of one or more of the many tendons and ligaments that surround the knee. The pain in these cases is not knee pain, strictly speaking, for it is from outside the joint.

Bone Spurs

Bone spurs are often demonstrated by X-ray and universally blamed for pain in the heel. In my experience, the spur is not symptomatic and the pain is usually due to TMS tendonalgia.

Soft Tissue Disorders: Fibromyalgia (Fibrositis, Myofibrositis, Myofasciitis)

Muscular rheumatism, chronic aches and pains, disturbed sleep, and morning stiffness affect a few million people in the United States, most of them women between the ages of twenty and fifty, and may be diagnosed as *fibromyalgia*. It is said that only a small percentage of fibromyalgia patients are properly diagnosed and that failing to find any laboratory abnormality, some doctors often conclude that the disorder is "psychogenic."

Though the diagnosis of fibromyalgia is being made with increasing frequency, the cause of the disorder is still said to be unknown. The patient is advised not to worry about it, because it's not "psychogenic" (putting it in quotes obviously means it's a bad word) and it is not degenerative or deforming.

For many years it has been clear to me that this disorder is one of the many variants of TMS. Therefore, though it is not degenerative or deforming, it certainly is psychogenic, for that is the overall term that covers a physical process that is induced by emotional factors. But, as has been said so many times in this book, many doctors have a visceral inability to accept such a concept. *Psychogenic* is a dirty word; it's what you call something if you can't figure out what it is. They cannot conceive of the possibility that emotions can cause bodily changes.

Doctors generally say they are not sure what causes fibromyalgia (TMS), but a laboratory abnormality has been identified in this disorder: it is oxygen deprivation, as noted in the physiology chapter (see page 72).

The trouble is that having identified a physiologic alteration, the doctors don't know what to do with the information, though they try mightily to explain it on physical and chemical grounds. With admirable erudition, they bring forth everything that is known about the physics and chemistry of muscle and with these facts construct an elaborate etiologic hypothesis, but the patient continues to be in pain.

Fibromyalgia is TMS. I have seen and treated hundreds of people with these symptoms over the years. As stated elsewhere, they suffer more severely than the average patient with TMS and often require psychotherapy.

Bursitis

A *bursa* is a structure designed to protect underlying bone in a place where there is a lot of pressure. There are two locations where pain is often attributed to an inflammation in the bursa: the shoulder and the hip. Medically, these are known as *subacromial bursitis* and *trochanteric bursitis*.

The shoulder is a complicated joint, and there are many things that may go wrong and cause pain. What I find most frequently is that the painful structure is a tendon passing above the bursa at or near the point of the tendon's attachment to bone (the acromion). Hence, the cause of the pain is a tendonalgia, not bursitis, and like most tendonalgias, is due to TMS. Thus, both the anatomy and the pathophysiology are wrong in many cases of TMS when the pain is attributed to subacromial bursitis.

Similarly, pain around what one might call the point of the hip (the trochanter) is usually ascribed to bursitis but in my experience is again a tendonalgia of TMS origin.

Tendon manifestations of TMS have been discussed in detail in other sections of the book and will be touched on briefly here.

Tendonitis

In the group of disorders referred to as *tendonitis,* the tendon is correctly identified as the offending part, but the reason given for the pain is incorrect. The anatomy is right, but the diagnosis is wrong. It is generally assumed that the painful tendon is inflamed because of overuse. So the treatment is to immobilize and rest the part and/or inject the tendon with a steroid (cortisone). Relief is often only temporary.

Many years ago, the suspicion dawned on me that tendonitis (more properly called *tendonalgia*) might be part of TMS when a patient reported that not only had his back pain resolved with treatment but also his elbow had ceased to hurt. I put this to the test and, indeed, found that I could get resolution of most tendonalgias. I now consider tendon/ligament to be the third type of tissue involved in TMS.

Common sites of tendonalgia are the shoulder, elbow, wrist, hip, knee, ankle, and foot.

Coccydynia

Coccydynia refers to pain deep in the midline crease between the buttocks. It is generally assumed that the tail end of the bone, the coccyx, is the source of pain, though it is quite clear that often the area involved is the lower end of the sacrum. Whether it is coccyx or sacrum, the symptom is usually a mystery to the diagnostician since nothing is seen on X-ray. Commonly, patients will relate it to a hard fall, usually in the distant past.

Coccydynia is a frequent manifestation of TMS and is probably a tendonalgia, since muscles attach to the sacrum and coccyx all along their length. Proof? It disappears with the talking treatment.

Neuroma

Another TMS tendonalgia attributed to something else is found in the fore part of the bottom of the foot. Pain is usually in the metatarsal region and is almost always blamed on a *neuroma,* which is a benign tumor. The pain goes with TMS treatment.

Plantar Fasciitis

The pain in *plantar fasciitis* is located on the bottom of the foot along the length of the arch. Although they are often vague about cause, doctors may ascribe this pain to inflammation. The area is usually very tender to palpation and seems quite clearly to be a manifestation of TMS.

Mononeuritis Multiplex

Mononeuritis multiplex is another descriptive diagnosis, for the cause is frequently unknown. It refers to nerve symptoms that appear to affect many nerves in a random pattern. It can occur with diabetes, but many people who have it are not diabetic. In my view, it is often an example of TMS neuralgia, because TMS tends to involve so many different muscles and nerves in the neck, shoulders, and back.

Temporomandibular Joint Syndrome (TMJ)

Temporomandibular joint syndrome is a very common, painful condition of the face that has historically been attributed to pathology of the jaw joint (TM joint) and, therefore, has been in the dental domain. I have never treated this disorder specifically but am strongly inclined to think that it is similar in cause to tension headache and TMS. TMS patients who come in for neck and shoulder pain frequently give a history of TMJ, and the jaw muscle is tender to palpation, just like the shoulder, back, and buttock muscles.

Inflammation

Inflammation must be discussed, for it is the explanation presented for many cases of upper and lower back pain and is the basis for the prescription of both steroidal (cortisone) and nonsteroidal (such as ibuprofen) anti-inflammatory drugs. Because of the magnitude of the back pain problem, these medications are widely used.

Experience with the diagnosis and treatment of TMS makes it clear that the source of the pain is neither spinal structures nor inflammation. An inflammatory process is an automatic reaction to disease or injury; it is basically a protective, healing process. The response to an invading bacteria or virus is an inflammation.

If that's what an inflammatory process is, what is going on in the back? Is it an infection, a response to a back injury—or what? No satisfactory, scientifically supported answer has ever been given. It has been suggested in this book that the source of the pain is oxygen deprivation and not inflammation. This idea has at least a modicum of support from the rheumatologic studies on fibromyalgia.

Sprain and Strain

The term *sprain* should be restricted to clear-cut instances of minor injury, like turning the ankle. I am not sure what a *strain* is supposed to be. Unfortunately, both of these terms are often used when the symptom is a TMS manifestation.

Having briefly reviewed these common traditional diagnoses for back pain, let us now look at the conventional treatments employed.

6

The Traditional (Conventional) Treatments

In a textbook chapter on the treatment of back pain, I once wrote that therapeutic eclecticism is a sign of diagnostic incompetence. The fact that there are so many different treatments for the common neck, shoulder, and back pain syndromes suggests that the diagnosticians are not really sure what the problem is. Of course, the patient is always given a diagnosis, usually a structural one, but subsequent management, including the use of medications, physical therapies of different kinds, manipulation, traction, acupuncture, biofeedback, transcutaneous nerve stimulation, and surgery, many of which are symptomatic treatments, suggests that the diagnoses are on shaky grounds.

People with TMS need to know about these treatments so they can understand why they did or did not respond to them or why they derived only partial or temporary benefit from them.

In thinking about how to review the subject, it occurred to me that the best approach might be to consider each treatment modality from the standpoint of its intended purpose. Of course, all treatments are supposed to relieve pain, but the important question is how. What is the rationale for each treatment? Before we get into this, let's review once more the subject of the placebo effect because of its crucial importance in any discussion of treatment.

THE PLACEBO EFFECT

A *placebo* is any treatment that produces a good therapeutic result despite the fact it has no intrinsic therapeutic value. A sugar pill is the classic example. It is clear that the desirable outcome must be attributed to the ability of the mind to manipulate the various organs and systems of the body. In order to do this, the mind must believe in the efficacy of the treatment and/or the treater. The key concept here is belief—the patient must have blind faith. But if he or she does, the result can be impressive. Consider the following story, which was first reported by Dr. Bruno Klopfer in 1957.

It concerns a man with a fulminating cancer of the lymph nodes who convinced his doctor to treat him with a drug called Krebiozen; the man had a miraculous recovery with disappearance of his many large tumors. He did well until he heard news reports of the ineffectiveness of Krebiozen, whereupon he regressed to the same desperate state in which he had been before.

Impressed with his response to the treatment, the doctor told him he would give him injections of a more powerful Krebiozen, but this time used only sterile water. Once more the patient responded dramatically, and his tumors melted away. When the American Medical Association officially announced the decision that Krebiozen was of no value, his tumors returned and he died soon after.

It is clear from this case history that a placebo works on the body not the imagination. In this instance, it stimulated a vigorous response in the immune system that was able to destroy the tumors.

Based on the impression that most of the pain syndromes I see are due to TMS, I have to conclude that beneficial results from most of the treatments to be described are the work of the placebo factor.

Treatments Designed to Rest an Injured Part

If the pain in a given case is truly the result of an injury, if some structure has been traumatized, if a period of healing is required, then treatments designed to rest an injured part are logical. They include rest in bed; the use of lumbar traction (which is really designed to keep the patient in bed, since the weights used could not possibly pull the spinal bones apart); restrictions on physical activity; and the use of cervical collars, lumbar corsets, or braces. The rest in bed is almost universally prescribed for patients thought to be suffering from a herniated disc.

If, however, there is no pathological structural abnormality, if the person has TMS, the rationale is gone. Not only are these prescriptions of no value but they also contribute to an intensification of the problem by suggesting to the patient that there is something going on dangerous enough to require complete immobilization. As emphasized in the treatment chapter, even the perception of a physical rather than an emotional cause for the pain will perpetuate the symptoms.

The collars and corsets used are a bit ridiculous, for they do not immobilize the part corseted. When someone reports feeling better or having become dependent on one of these, I think *placebo*.

Treatments to Relieve Pain

Pain relief is the goal of all treatments, but treatments to relieve pain are designed to take away pain per se. Generally, this is symptomatic treatment and, therefore, poor medicine unless it is administered for humanitarian purposes. The use of morphine, Demerol, or other strong analgesics is certainly justified when there is excruciating pain but not as a definitive treatment.

Acupuncture appears to work as a local anesthetic. In other words, it blocks the transmission of pain nerve impulses to the brain. If one is dealing with a chronic disease for which no relief of pain can be expected, this is a good treatment. For the typical back patient, it can give temporary relief but it does nothing about the underlying process, the cause of the pain.

Nerve blocks are widely used across the country, especially when pain is severe and intractable. A local anesthetic is injected and does essentially what acupuncture does. Therefore, the criticism of this as treatment for back pain is the same.

Transcutaneous nerve stimulation (TNS) depends on mild electric shocks administered over the painful area to give pain relief. Electrodes are usually taped in place, and the patient can activate the shock at will. One can say the same thing about this as for the two above. However, there is a real question whether this functions as anything but a placebo. A group at the Mayo Clinic published a study in 1978 in which they demonstrated that a placebo worked equally well (G. Thorsteinsson, H. H. Stonnington, G. K. Stillwell, and L. R. Elveback, "The Placebo Effect of Transcutaneous Electrical Stimulation," *Pain*, Vol. 5, p. 31).

When there is prolonged relief as a result of any of these treatments, one must suspect a placebo effect; there can be no other explanation, for they do not attack the cause of the problem.

Treatments to Promote Relaxation

To the prescribers of treatments to promote relaxation, I would put the question, "To what end?" "What is your purpose in trying to relax the person?" "What do you hope to accomplish?"

There is considerable fuzziness about this subject in the area of pain relief. There is no question that a calm, relaxed person will experience less pain, but again we are engaged in symptomatic treatment. The basic disorder is not being treated. And how much time can be devoted each day to the relaxing exercises? I advise my patients that meditation and relaxation exercises can't hurt, but one cannot depend on them for definitive relief of pain.

The specific role of *biofeedback* in pain relief is to produce muscle relaxation. The usual procedure is to affix small electrodes over forehead muscles whose electrical activity (which reflects muscular activity) then registers on a gauge or screen. The subject is then instructed to reduce the gauge reading, which means the muscle has relaxed and this in turn produces reflex relaxation in muscles elsewhere in the body.

I do not prescribe biofeedback, as, again, it is treating the symptom.

Treatments to Correct a Structural Abnormality

Probably the most common treatment among those used to correct a structural abnormality is *manipulation*. The abnormality for which this is used is malalignment of spinal bones, and the purpose of treatment is to restore alignment. I do not believe the abnormality exists, and if it did, I do not believe it could be changed by manipulation. On occasion, dramatic relief of pain follows a manipulation, suggesting that the person is having a good placebo response. Patients generally return for these treatments regularly. It is likely, therefore, that they are having a placebo response, which is known to be temporary.

Though not as common as manipulation, *surgery* to remove extruded intervertebral disc material is frequently performed. Without question, such procedures are often essential. It is my impression, however, based upon my experience with patients with herniated discs, that the extruded disc material is often not responsible for the pain. Needless to say, the physicians who perform these operations do so with the sincere conviction that an offending substance is being removed; this is the concept that governs the decision to do surgery, and it is widely held. Nevertheless, because of my therapeutic experience, I am forced to the conclusion that surgery may sometimes produce a desirable result because of the placebo effect. The strength of a placebo, meaning its ability to achieve a good and permanent effect, is measured by the impression it makes on the person's mind. This is why surgery is probably a very powerful placebo.

That fact was brought to the attention of the medical world in 1961 ("Surgery as a Placebo," *Journal of the American Medical Association*, Vol. 176, p. 1102) by the same Henry Beecher who reported on the reactions of men wounded in battle (see chapter 7 on the mind and body). One hesitates to impugn the value of surgery, but there is considerable anecdotal evidence of its failure in many cases. As has been stated throughout this book, TMS rather than disc herniation appears to be the cause of pain in most cases. Therefore, the removal of herniated disc material may not address the basic problem.

There is another treatment that might be characterized as pseudosurgical, since its purpose, as with surgery, is to remove herniated disc material. *Chymopapain* is an enzyme that can be injected into the extruded toothpaste-like disc material and will digest (dissolve) it. This procedure is less formidable than an operation but must bear the same criticism as surgery since the herniated disc material may not be the cause of pain. Further, serious reactions to this enzyme have been reported in the medical literature.

Cervical traction, which can actually distract (pull apart) the cervical bones to a slight degree, is another attempt to alter a structural abnormality—in this case to try to make the cervical foramina larger. These are the holes formed by two spinal bones through which the spinal nerves make their way. The idea is to make the holes larger so the nerves won't be "pinched." But we have said before that the idea that they are being pinched is usually fantasy, and, once again, there is much ado about nothing.

Treatments to Strengthen Muscles

For years the doctrine of strengthening back and abdominal muscles to protect the back or relieve it of pain has been preached across the length and breadth of the land. It is an idea that is deeply ingrained in the American mind—and it is dead wrong. Programs are taught in the YMCA, exercise is prescribed by thousands of doctors, and people are trained by a large variety of therapists.

There is nothing wrong with doing these exercises and strengthening these muscles; it's a very good thing (I do them myself). But, I tell my patients, they will neither make your pain go away nor protect you from it, and if they do, you are having a placebo effect.

What about using exercise to get you going, to break your fear of physical activity? That is a very different story and a very good use for exercise.

Dr. Hubert Rosomoff, mentioned in connection with his repudiation of the significance of disc pathology, has a large, successful program for the conservative treatment of persistent pain syndromes associated with the School of Medicine in Miami, Florida. His program of physical activity is both vigorous and rigorous from all reports. It is my impression, however, that though his patients improve and become more functional, many continue to have pain. From my point of view, this is inevitable since the basic cause of the disorder has not been identified and addressed.

Only very occasionally will I refer a patient to a physical therapist and then only for help in overcoming fear and reluctance to do physical exercise.

Treatments to Increase Local Circulation of Blood

There are a number of physical treatments that will increase the flow of blood into an area by increasing the temperature of the tissue. Heat can be generated within muscle, for example, by the use of *shortwave* or *ultrasonic radiation*. *Deep massage* and *active exercise* will do the same thing. Contrary to what one might expect, a *hot pack* will not increase blood flow, since the heat does not penetrate the skin, let alone reach the muscle. Paradoxically, an *ice pack* may increase it by stimulating a reflex response to the cold.

But what does one accomplish by doing this? Unless the pain is somehow the result of decreased blood flow or reduced oxygenation resulting from some other mechanism, increasing available oxygen is of no value.

As the reader is aware, it is our hypothesis, now supported by rheumatology research, that oxygen deprivation is precisely the mechanism of TMS muscle pain. Nevertheless, I do not use these therapeutic modalities, because they are only of temporary value and because they are physical. The rationale for this decision was discussed at length in the chapter on the treatment of TMS.

The application of hot or cold packs, the use of radiation (these days mostly ultrasonic), deep and superficial massage, and active exercise are widely used in the treatment of pain syndromes, almost regardless of presumed etiology. For example, a diagnosis of herniated disc is made, but it is decided that surgery is not warranted. In that case, after a period of rest in bed, physical therapy will often be prescribed if pain continues, usually consisting of deep heat, massage, and exercise. It is difficult to understand what this is intended to do. It will not change the anatomical status of the extruded disc material. It will temporarily increase blood flow and may tone up muscles, but to what end?

As one who wrote this prescription perhaps thousands of times many years ago, I must confess that the rationale was often fuzzy and there was not a little wishful thinking involved: "Do something, and maybe the pain will go away," "Strengthen the abdominal and back muscles to support the spine," "Relax the muscles," and so forth.

If the physical therapist was particularly talented, the results were often very good. Alas, here again was the placebo response at work, meaning that the result was usually not permanent. However, if the therapist remained available to the patient, another round of therapy might result in pain relief for a few more weeks or months. But the patient continued to live a life circumscribed by many prohibitions and admonitions and the always present fear of a recurrence of pain.

Treatments to Combat Inflammation

My immediate response to any treatment to combat inflammation is, "What inflammation?" To the best of my knowledge, no one has ever demonstrated the existence of an inflammatory process in any back pain syndrome, and yet enormous amounts of steroidal and nonsteroidal anti-inflammatory medication are used in treatment, both pre-scription and nonprescription. Judging the efficacy of these drugs is a bit difficult, because most of them have analgesic (painkilling) abilities as well. Since there is no inflammation in TMS, one must assume that improvement with these is due either to their painkilling function or placebo effect.

With one exception. Steroids (so-called cortisone drugs) will reduce or banish the symptoms of TMS temporarily in many patients. I do not know how or why this happens. I see these people when the pain returns; they have TMS—and they usually respond to treatment with permanent resolution of symptoms.

TREATING CHRONIC PAIN

Near the end of chapter 4 on the treatment of TMS, I described a program that is in wide use across the country to treat *chronic pain*. It bears repeating here that treating pain is not medically sound. Pain is a symptom, like fever. It has been elevated to the status of a separate disorder on the hypothesis that certain psychological factors cause the patient to exaggerate the pain. As stated before, this theory requires that one acknowledge the continuing presence of a structural reason for the pain—which is then exaggerated.

In my experience, in both the mild and the severe, the acute and the chronic pain syndromes, in the majority of patients it is the physiologic changes characteristic of TMS that are responsible for the pain and not a structural abnormality. These physiologic alterations result in pain and other symptoms. To treat those symptoms is no wiser than treating the fever in someone with pneumococcal pneumonia.

Where did this new theory come from? The problem originated with the failure of physicians to accurately diagnose the reason for the pain. Then, when it became severe, chronic, and disabling, they threw up their hands and hoped that someone would relieve them of the burden of caring for these patients. Physicians were happy to shift the responsibility when the behavioral psychologists came along with the theory that psychological needs created a brand-new disorder that they called *chronic pain*. Pain was elevated to the status of a disease by psychological fiat when frustrated physicians abrogated their appropriate role as diagnosticians.

Pain is, has been, and always will be a symptom. If it becomes severe and chronic, it is because that which is causing it is severe and has gone unrecognized. Chronicity, in the case of these pain syndromes, is a function of faulty diagnosis. The following case history makes this clear and is a fitting conclusion for this chapter.

The patient was a middle-aged woman with a grown-up family; she had been essentially bedridden for about two years when she came to our attention. She had suffered from low back and leg pain for years, had been operated on twice, and had gradually deteriorated to the point where her life was restricted almost entirely to her upstairs bedroom.

She was admitted to the hospital where we found no evidence of a continuing structural problem but severe manifestations of TMS. And no wonder, for the psychological evaluation revealed that she had endured terrible sexual and psychological abuse as a child and that she was in a rage, to put it mildly, and had no awareness of it. She was a pleasant, motherly sort of woman, the kind that would automatically repress anger. And so it festered in her for years, always kept in check by the severe pain syndrome.

Her recovery was stormy, for as the details of her life came out and she began to acknowledge her fury, she experienced a variety of physical symptoms—cardiocirculatory, gastrointestinal, allergic—but the pain began to recede. Group and individual psychotherapy was intense. Fortunately, she was very intelligent and grasped the concepts of TMS quickly. As the pain reduced, the staff helped to get her mobile again. Fourteen weeks after admission, she went home essentially free of pain and ready to resume her life again.

This woman did not have the disease "chronic pain." She had a physical disorder, TMS, induced by fearful psychological trauma. What a disservice to her if it had been implied that her pain was so great and persistent because she was deriving psychological benefit from it. Thus, just one example of why I am opposed to this concept.

And as well, my insistence that the treatment of TMS requires an educational-psychotherapeutic approach. Most patients do not need psychotherapy, but they do need to know that all of us generate and repress bad feelings and that these feelings may be the cause of physical symptoms.

7

Mind and Body

One thing that is abundantly clear about the cause and treatment of TMS is that it is a striking example of what might be called the mind-body connection. The history of medicine's awareness of this interaction is long and checkered. Hippocrates advised his asthmatic patients to be wary of anger, which suggests that 2,500 years ago there was some appreciation of the impact of the emotions on illness. That concept was dealt a crippling blow by the seventeenth-century philosopher and mathematician René Descartes, who held that the mind and body were totally separate entities and should be studied separately. Matters of the mind were the concern of religion and philosophy, according to Descartes. The body, he said, should be studied by objective, verifiable methods. To a large extent, Descartes's teaching remains the model for contemporary medical research and practice. The average physician looks upon illness as a disorder of the body machine and sees his role as discovering the nature of the defect and correcting it. Research in medicine rests heavily on the laboratory, and what cannot be studied in the laboratory is widely considered to be unscientific. Despite the obvious fallacy of that idea, it remains the guiding research principle for most medical investigators. The spirit of Descartes is still very much alive.

CHARCOT AND FREUD

In the late nineteenth century, the famous French neurologist Jean-Martin Charcot gave new life to the principle of the interacting mind and body when he shared with the medical world his experiences with a group of intriguing patients. Called *hysterics,* they had dramatic neurological symptoms, like paralysis of an arm or leg, with no evidence of neurological disease. Imagine the effect on his medical audience, however, when he demonstrated that the paralysis could be made to disappear when the patient was hypnotized! One could not ask for a more convincing demonstration of the mind-body connection.

Among the many physicians who came to Charcot's famous clinics was a Viennese neurologist, Sigmund Freud. His name is now a household word, as well it should be, for he developed the concept of the unconscious mind (subconscious, if you wish), without which it would be impossible to understand human behavior. However, despite the fact that Freud began to write on this subject about one hundred years ago, awareness of subconscious emotional activity and its effect on what people do and how they feel is still largely limited to analytically trained psychiatrists and psychologists. This is particularly unfortunate, since disorders like TMS, peptic ulcer, and colitis originate in

156

the subconscious and have to do with emotions that are generated there.

Freud became intensely interested in patients with hysteria and began to work with them. He was motivated by the observation that hypnosis might banish the symptom temporarily, but it did not cure. Eventually Freud concluded that the dramatic pseudosymptoms exhibited by these patients, which he called *conversion hysterical symptoms,* were the result of a complicated subconscious process in which painful emotions were repressed and then discharged physically. He thought that the symptoms were symbolic and represented a discharge of emotional tension. It was his idea that the process of repression was a defense against the painful emotions. He made a distinction, however, between the kind of symptoms these patients had and those that affected the internal organs, like the stomach and colon. He believed the latter fell into a different category and could not be treated psychologically. He found that he was able to help many of the conversion hysterical patients through the therapeutic process of psychoanalysis, which he developed and for which he has become justly famous.

In my view, Freud's greatest contribution to medicine was his recognition of the existence of the human unconscious and his continuous efforts to understand it throughout his career. His accomplishments stand with those of Einstein, Galileo, and other great, innovative scientists.

FRANZ ALEXANDER

Though Freud may be said to have been the first great proponent of the mind-body connection, and though he remained interested in the subject all his life, it was his students who made the greatest contributions to the field. Perhaps the most important of these was Franz Alexander, who, with his colleagues at the Institute for Psychoanalysis in Chicago, did some of the most important work of this century in the field of psychosomatic medicine. He moved beyond Freud in this field by asserting that organ abnormalities, like peptic ulcer, were also induced by psychological phenomena, though different from those that caused conversion hysterical symptoms. What he called a vegetative neurosis (like ulcers and colitis) he said was a physiologic response to constant or recurring emotional states. He studied disorders of the upper and lower gastrointestinal tracts, bronchial asthma, cardiac arrhythmias, high blood pressure, psychogenic and migraine headache, skin disorders, diabetes, hyperthyroidism, and rheumatoid arthritis. In each case, he thought there was a specific psychological situation that mandated that particular disorder; for example, suppressed rage would produce high blood pressure. (I shall return to this concept later on page 169 when I explain my theories on the causation of psychologically induced physical disorders.)

Alexander made another important contribution by reviewing the history of medical psychology (in *Psychosomatic Medicine*, New York: Norton, 1950) and pointing out that with the advent of modern scientific medicine in the nineteenth century, the study of the impact of psychology on health and illness was abandoned. Modern medicine believed that everything could be explained on the basis of physics and chemistry, that the body was an incredibly complicated machine, and all you had to do was learn how it was put together, how it reacted to attacks upon it, and you could create perfect health and freedom from disease. As was said above, this idea was first promulgated by Descartes and was a reaction to medicine's spiritual and mystical past. Therefore, medical science looked down on Freud and his followers and accused them of being unscientific.

THE DOMINANCE OF THE PHYSICOCHEMICAL CONCEPT OF PATHOLOGY

Alexander thought that he had successfully met the criticisms of the medical scientific community by employing rigorous scientific methods in his work and proclaimed that we were now about to enter a new era in medicine in which the role of the emotions in health and illness would be appreciated and vigorously studied. But alas, it was not to be. As Freud's enthusiastic and talented pupils disappeared from the medical scene, so did the concept that emotions were directly responsible for certain medical disorders and played an important role in others. The Cartesian medical philosophers once more established their dominance, and the emotions were banished from the field of medical research. The medical journal *Psychosomatic Medicine,* established by Alexander and his colleagues, was taken over by workers whose primary interests were the laboratory and statistics. If it couldn't be studied in the laboratory, they said, it wasn't "scientific," ergo the mind-body idea was unscientific and couldn't be studied.

As the years went by, the physical-chemical view of medicine became so strong that a substantial number of psychiatrists began to call themselves *biological psychiatrists,* proclaiming that emotional ills were the result of chemical abnormalities of brain function and that all that one had to do was discover the nature of the chemical defect in each disorder and then correct it with a pharmaceutical product. According to them, depression and anxiety are simply derangements of brain chemicals. Naturally, the developers and purveyors of pharmaceuticals were delighted with this turn of events, but they did not initiate it—the psychiatric community did.

The obvious fallacy of this kind of thinking is that there are undoubtedly chemical changes that can be detected in the brain associated with both normal and "abnormal" emotional states but that the chemistry is not the cause but the mechanics or result of the emotional state. If you treat the patient with chemicals, you are practicing poor medicine by treating the symptom rather than the cause.

For instance, Mr. Jones is anxious because he is facing financial reverses, and he is having a variety of anxiety symptoms. His doctor gives him a tranquilizer rather than suggesting something that will help him to deal with the realities of his situation. This is poor medicine.

The swing back to a predominantly physicochemical view of pathology has happened in the last thirty-five years. At this moment, mainstream medicine seems to be far away from showing any interest in mind-body relationships. As recently as June 1985, an editorial writer for the *New England Journal of Medicine,* one of our most prestigious publications, wrote that most of what is known about this subject is folklore. The editorial brought a storm of protest from around the world, because good research is beginning to be done in this field. But it demonstrated the confidence and arrogance of the loyal followers of Descartes. Fortunately, some balance was provided by an equally important medical journal, a British one, the *Lancet,* the following month, July 1985, when its editorial writer commented on the work that was being done in the field of mind-body relationships and suggested that the medical community might begin to pay greater attention to it. The editorial wasn't a ringing endorsement for research in this area, but it was certainly more objective and scientific than the *New England Journal* editorial.

THE CURRENT STATUS OF MIND-BODY RESEARCH

If I have painted a grim picture, it is because the overwhelming majority of clinical work and research in the United States continues to be structurally oriented. There are, however, some bright spots, so all is not lost. New ideas always have rough sledding and are generally rejected when first presented, particularly if they challenge or go beyond principles that have been cherished and fruitful for a long time. The most dramatic and valuable advances in medicine in the last one hundred years have been the result of laboratory discoveries (such as penicillin), and we owe a great debt to what might be called the era of laboratory medicine. But we must be able to move forward and realize that new methods of research may be necessary, particularly if one engages to study something as difficult and mysterious as the mind.

Franz Alexander quotes Einstein as having said that Aristotle's ideas of motion retarded the development of mechanics for two thousand years (also in *Psychosomatic Medicine*). It would be a pity if Cartesian philosophy were to do the same thing to the study of the influence of the mind, particularly the emotions, on the body.

Why do contemporary physicians have trouble with mind-body concepts? I believe it is because they see themselves as engineers to the human body. According to them, health and illness can be expressed in physical and chemical terms, and the idea that a thought or an emotion could somehow have an effect on that physicochemistry is anathema. This is why my work has been so studiously ignored. I have demonstrated conclusively that a truly physical-pathological process is the result of emotional phenomena and can be halted by a mental one. That is, first of all, rank heresy, and secondly, beyond the comprehension of most physicians. Nothing in their training prepared them for such an idea, and to them it smacks of voodoo. It reminds them, with a shudder, of the old era of unscientific medicine before Descartes. Paradoxically, thoughtful laymen are much more able to accept such an idea, because they are not burdened with a medical education and all the philosophical biases that go along with it. Contemporary medical science is scientifically limited, because it has closed itself off from further progress, being unwilling to venture out beyond the secure boundaries of its familiar technology. It ought to take a lesson from the field of theoretical physics where old ideas are constantly being revised in the light of new knowledge.

MY HYPOTHESES ON THE NATURE OF MIND-BODY INTERACTIONS

Before reviewing recent progress in our understanding of mind-body interactions, it might be well to describe my hypotheses bearing on this subject. Most of these ideas have developed as a result of my experience in the diagnosis and treatment of TMS. I emphasize that they are hypothetical.

The first, and most basic, idea is that mental and emotional states can impinge upon and alter, for good or ill, any of the body's organs or systems. The mechanism by which this is accomplished is unknown to us, though research is beginning to suggest answers. But that should not disturb us, for no more can we explain how it is that the brain can take the jumble of sounds that enter our ears and turn them into comprehensible words or the myriad shapes and lines we see with the eyes that mean nothing until the brain has worked on them and converted them into words or things we recognize. Most of what the brain does (all subconsciously) is a complete mystery to us. Why, then, are we disturbed because we can't explain how mental and emotional phenomena can do things to the brain and the body? Things that happen at Lourdes are real; things that Indian fakirs do are real; the placebo

163

effect is real. It is the job of medical science to study rather than scoff at them.

Let me emphasize that in my view, the mind can influence *any* physical process.

The Composition of the Psyche

For almost a hundred years, it has been appreciated that the makeup of the emotional structure of the mind, what one might call the psyche, is multifaceted. The psyche appears to be composed of multiple, sometimes conflicting forces, and they function primarily below the level of consciousness. We owe this knowledge largely to Freud, who worked all his life to understand and describe them. His formulations and descriptions of id, ego, and superego are well known. I do not possess the background or knowledge required to do a psychoanalytic analysis of my observations. What I can do is describe what I have seen, present my impressions of what it means psychologically, and leave it to the experts to decide where these observations fit in contemporary psychoanalytic theory.

To make things easy, we can refer to this multifaceted emotional mechanism as the *personality*. We all have one, and we are all aware of some of its characteristics; for example, we know if we're compulsive or perfectionistic. But there are important components of our personalities that we are unaware of, that are in the unconscious, that may have a profound effect on our lives. It seems clear that all human beings possess the same basic parts of the personality structure, though there may be considerable variation in the composition of these parts and the relative importance of each part in the life of the individual. For example, everyone has a conscience; in one person it may be so strong as to virtually dominate his life; in the next so weak that his social behavior borders on the criminal.

A very important part of the unconscious personality is that which is childish, primitive, and, therefore, narcissistic. It is self-involved, to the exclusion of concern for the needs, desires, and comforts of others. It is me oriented. The size (strength, influence) of this part varies from person to person. In some people it is large, and they are, therefore, more liable to react or behave in self-indulgent or childish ways, though the latter may be hard to detect since people's demeanor is always papered over by adult behavior. Many feelings and behaviors are no doubt left over from childhood. Children feel weak and vulnerable; they are dependent, and they feel that dependency strongly; they don't think much of themselves; they have a constant need for approval; they are very prone to anxiety and quick to anger. They have no patience. To a degree, we all continue to generate some of those feelings unconsciously right on into adulthood. What varies from person to person is how much.

Joseph Campbell, the great mythologist, philosopher, and teacher, taught that primitive tribes had rites of passage, by which boys and girls became men and women. They were always dramatic, often traumatic, and always specific and powerful. No doubt they helped diminish the influence of the residual child by making a sharp demarcation between childhood and adulthood. Modern, "civilized" society has no such rites (the Bar Mitzvah and confirmation come closest, but they are certainly not as powerful), and it may be that we suffer from the lack of them. If the line between childhood and adulthood is blurred, we may retain more of our childish tendencies despite chronological age.

It is possible that the anxiety that is a part of everyone's life stems from the response of this part of our emotional systems to the stresses and strains of daily existence. The greater the stress, the more anxiety is generated. And, as stated in the psychology chapter, the same goes for anger.

Anger may be one of the most important and least appreciated of the emotions we generate. The celebrated psychoanalyst and ethicist Willard Gaylin published a book in 1984 titled *The Rage Within,* which explored the subject of anger in modern man. Because anger is so antithetical to our idea of appropriate behavior in a civilized society, we tend to repress it at the very moment it is generated in the unconscious and so remain unaware of its existence. There are many reasons, most of them unconscious, why we repress anger. They were enumerated in the psychology chapter (see page 45).

The tendency to *repress* undesirable emotions is a supremely important element of one's emotional life, and, again, we are indebted to Freud for the concept. We repress feelings of anxiety, anger, weakness, dependency, and low self-esteem, for obvious reasons.

At the other end of the emotional spectrum, there is what Freud called the superego; this is our Moses. It tells us what we should and should not be doing, and it can be a hard taskmaster. In fact, it adds to the pressures that make us anxious and angry and so actually contributes to the tensions within us. As I have said earlier, people who get TMS tend to be hardworking, hyper-responsible, conscientious, ambitious, and achieving, all of which build up the pressure on the beleaguered self.

One further observation. Just as there is a powerful tendency to repress undesirable emotions, there seems to be an equally strong drive to bring them to consciousness. It is this threat to overcome repression that necessitates the creation by the brain of such things as TMS, ulcers, and migraines.

TMS as an Example of Mind-Body Interaction: The Principle of Equivalence

We can now proceed to an examination of the question of where TMS fits into the broader mind-body scheme. It is certainly a prime example of such a reaction. I see it as one of a group of physical reactions, all generated for the same purpose. TMS is equivalent to peptic ulcer, spastic colitis, constipation, tension headache, migraine headache, cardiac palpitations, eczema, allergic rhinitis (hay fever), prostatitis (often), ringing in the ears (often), and dizziness (often). This is a partial list but represents the most common of such reactions. Anecdotally, I have seen laryngitis, pathological dry mouth, frequent urination, and many others serving the same purpose. I believe these disorders are interchangeable and equivalents of each other, because many of them are found to occur historically in patients with TMS, sometimes at the same time, but often in tandem. I recently saw a patient who reported that he had been having severe migraine headaches (probably tension headaches from his description), but ever since his low back pain and sciatica came on, the headaches had ceased.

Equivalence is also suggested by the fact that patients often report resolution of one of these disorders when the TMS pain goes away. This happens most commonly with hay fever. I teach **patients** that all the conditions on the list serve the same **purpose** psychologically.

Consider the **following** excerpt from a letter I received just a few months **ago.** The man first wrote that his wife, a back pain patient, was doing very nicely. And then this:

"You may remember that after the lecture I approached you and mentioned that I had been suffering from stomach problems for the past twenty years. You told me that the same principle applied. Well to my disbelief it worked! I had been taking pills of all sorts and Maalox for years— more years than I'd like to admit. My stomach problems had started in my third year of high school. I was unable to eat a meal without the immediate need to take some kind of stomach medication or another. By applying your theory and realizing how much the subconscious mind controls our everyday living, my stomach problems have completely gone away. Nobody believes me when I try to explain it to them but I'm sure you understand."

You can be sure no one believes him, for laymen generally take their cues from the medical profession on health matters, and we have already described medicine's position on such things. It is my judgment that only 10 percent of the population would understand that man's experience.

From a theoretical point of view, there are some interesting implications suggested by this equivalence principle. As far as the group of disorders I have listed is concerned, it deviates from Franz Alexander's hypothesis that specific disorders have particular psychological significance. In his classic book, he discussed the psychodynamics he thought responsible for gastrointestinal, respiratory, and cardiovascular problems. Experience with TMS and these related conditions suggests that there may be a common denominator, anxiety perhaps, that can bring on any one of these disorders. In that case, some other emotion, anger, for example, may be the primary one that may in turn induce anxiety, which then brings on the symptom.

Personally, I have experienced gastric hyperacidity, colitis, migraine headache, palpitations, and a variety of musculoskeletal symptoms typical of TMS and know that they were all the result of repressed anger. Once having learned the trick, I could usually identify the reason for the anger—and often turn off the symptom.

It is interesting to note that most of the disorders listed above are mediated through the autonomic nervous system. As far as we know, hay fever is not but represents malfunction in the immune system. I shall return to this later when we discuss the new field of psychoneuroimmunology (see page 174).

The Physical Disorder as a Defense Against Repressed Emotions

This has been discussed in chapter 2 on psychology, and it will be only briefly reiterated here that the purpose of the physical symptomatology, whether it is musculoskeletal, gastrointestinal, or genitourinary, is to distract attention, which is a mechanism for allowing the individual to avoid feeling or dealing with the undesirable emotions, whatever they may be. It is, in essence, a lack of desire of the mind to cope with these feelings. One must make a sharp distinction, however, between a decision made in the subconscious and one that the person would consciously make. As pointed out earlier in the book, TMS patients cope only too well in reality; it is their unconscious minds that are cowardly. The best evidence of the validity of this concept is the fact that patients are able to stop the process simply by *learning about it*. The diversion (distraction) no longer works when it is identified for what it is. As mentioned in chapter 4 on treatment, many people have reported resolution of their back pain syndromes after reading my first book, making it quite clear that they were "cured" by the acquired information. That could not be a placebo.

Freud and his students recognized that hysterical symptoms sometimes took the form of pain. Over the years, I have seen a number of patients with severe manifestations of TMS, so severe that they were usually bedridden. In addition to having the classic findings of TMS—that is, pain on pressure over certain muscles and involvement of nerves like the sciatic—these patients often had pain in strange locations and of a bizarre quality. "I feel as though there is cracked glass under my skin" is a typical example. Freud would have called this hysterical pain. Hysterical symptoms involve the sensorimotor system instead of the autonomic, which is what distinguishes them from gastrointestinal symptoms, for example, and suggests that they have a different psychological cause. It is my view that both TMS and its equivalents and so-called hysterical pain stem from the same source psychologically but that the magnitude of the emotional problem may determine which symptoms the brain chooses.

A Unitary Theory of
Psychologically Induced Pain

In July 1959, Dr. Allan Walters delivered a presidential address to the eleventh annual meeting of the Canadian Neurological Society titled "Psychogenic Regional Pain Alias Hysterical Pain." The address was published in the journal *Brain* in March 1961. It was Dr. Walters's contention that the designation of hysterical pain was not accurate, since in his experience a large variety of mental and nervous states could induce the kind of pain usually identified as hysterical, and not just hysteria. (Note the similarity to what I have just proposed above.) Typical of hysterical pain, it occurred in locations that did not make neuroanatomical sense.

Walters proposed the term *psychogenic regional pain* for this kind of pain. *Psychogenic* because it was clearly the result of a mental or emotional disorder. (All of the patients had been thoroughly studied to rule out physical lesions.) *Regional,* because the pain involved a particular region of the body without regard to specific nerve distributions.

My experience supports and extends Dr. Walters's observations. I have seen either the pain of TMS, which includes muscle, nerve, tendon, or ligament pain, or psychogenic regional pain in patients with anxiety states of varying degrees of severity as well as in patients with schizophrenia and manic-depressive conditions. It appears that the brain will choose from a large repertoire of painful and nonpainful disorders when it needs to defend against painful or undesirable feelings. We usually see the regional pain when the emotional state is severe.

I would further hypothesize that in addition to varying degrees of severity of the emotional disorder (for example, mild, moderate, or severe anxiety), individuals repress these feelings to different levels. One has the impression that in some people these feelings are so deeply buried that it becomes difficult to impossible for the psychotherapist to get the patient to bring them to consciousness. In others the feelings are just below the surface. Undoubtedly, those that are most painful and/or frightening are more deeply buried.

In my practice, patients with more severe problems, usually requiring psychotherapy in addition to the educational program, account for about 5 percent of those I see.

The Emotions and More Serious Disorders

There are those in medicine who believe that emotions play a role in all aspects of health and illness. I am one of them. Alexander suggested doing away with the term *psychosomatic medicine* since it was redundant—everything medical is influenced in some way by the emotions. I believe that all medical studies are flawed if they do not consider the emotional factor. For example, a research project dealing with hardening of the arteries usually includes consideration of diet (cholesterol), weight, exercise, genetic factors—but if it does not include emotional factors, the results, in my view, are not valid.

Before discussing other kinds of medical problems in which emotions may play a prominent role, it is important to make it clear that people do not do these things to themselves. It is not uncommon for patients to say to me after the diagnosis of TMS has been made, "I feel terrible; I did it to myself." Upon which I tell them that their emotional patterns were well established long before they reached the age of responsibility and that what they are now is a result of a combination of genetic and developmental-environmental factors over which they had no control. Might as well take responsibility for how tall you are or the color of your eyes. Therefore, they are reacting to life in the only way they know how. Further, if one begins to understand why one reacts the way one does and wants to change, some degree of progress is possible.

Another reaction of a similar nature is that of physicians who resist acknowledging the role of emotions—in cancer, for example. They say it is cruel to suggest to patients that emotions may have contributed to the onset of the cancer; it makes them feel guilty and responsible. My answer to this is that it makes a world of difference how you introduce the subject to patients. You don't bludgeon them with the information and make it sound as though they are emotionally defective. You explain that they are not responsible as described above and talk to them about their lives, try to identify emotional factors that might have contributed to the cancer process, and then follow it up with concrete suggestions as to how they can remedy and reverse the negative factors. I do not mean to suggest that there is a well-worked-out therapeutic process in existence based on such ideas. This is an area in which a great deal of research must be done.

THE CURRENT STATE OF THE ART OF MIND-BODY MEDICINE

Readers who are interested in an excellent review of where medicine is today vis-à-vis the mind-body connection should read *The Healer Within* by Steven Locke, MD, and Douglas Colligan (New York: Dutton, 1986). Dr. Locke is in the Department of Psychiatry at Harvard Medical School and has done an excellent job with his writer-collaborator describing the history and contemporary efforts to understand how the mind influences the body.

There is nothing important in the book with which I disagree. However, I have the impression that the authors focus too heavily on the immune system and imply that the future of this field depends upon what they call the "science of psychoneuroimmunology." The study of psychoneuroimmunology is highly scientific and will play an important role in our understanding of many serious disorders, such as cancer and the autoimmune diseases (like rheumatoid arthritis and diabetes), but in my view it is but one segment of a larger study of how emotions may influence any of the organs and systems of the body.

TMS is an example of a mind-body disorder mediated through the autonomic nervous system; the immune system is not involved. I suspect the immune system does not participate in the interaction of emotions and the cardiovascular system. Once more, one is intrigued by the fact that the brain crosses boundaries in responding to its psychological needs. Thus, patients with the same psychological diagnosis (though differing in severity) may develop TMS, autonomically mediated; allergic rhinitis,

174

immune system mediated; or psychogenic regional pain, direct action on the sensorimotor system.

Extremely important work is being done in the brain biochemistry section of the National Institutes of Mental Health on the subject of brain-body interaction. One of the pioneers in this research is Candace Pert, once chief of that section, whose work is demonstrating communication between the brain and different parts and systems of the body. For those interested, an excellent review of this work appeared in the June 1989 issue of *Smithsonian,* written by Stephen S. Hall.

The mind and body interact in numerous ways; the following part of the chapter reviews some of those more common interactions.

MIND AND THE CARDIOVASCULAR SYSTEM

The subjects of interest to us in the category of the mind and the cardiovascular system are hypertension, coronary artery disease, arteriosclerosis (hardening of the arteries), cardiac palpitations, and mitral valve prolapse.

High blood pressure (hypertension), as everyone knows, is very common and a little scary because of its connection with heart trouble and stroke. Its association with emotions has been assumed by many, though never demonstrated in the laboratory. Dr. Neal Miller, a psychologist working at Rockefeller University, demonstrated that laboratory animals could be conditioned to lower their blood pressure and modify many other bodily processes, too, clearly showing that the brain could be recruited to influence the body.

Dr. Herbert Benson, a Harvard cardiologist, has described what he calls the relaxation response and demonstrated that the blood pressure can be reduced by the application of this meditation-like process.

A very important study appeared in the *Journal of the American Medical Association* in the April 11, 1990, issue (Vol. 263, pp. 1929–35). Dr. Peter L. Schnall and a team from the Cardiovascular and Hypertension Center, New York Hospital–Cornell Medical College, in collaboration with doctors from two other New York area medical schools, published a paper that established a clear relationship between psychological pressure at work ("job strain") and high blood pressure. The study also established the fact that there was an increase in the size of the heart in these people, which is one of the undesirable effects of sustained hypertension. Experts have long suspected that psychological factors were implicated in high blood pressure. The great value of Dr. Schnall's study is that it was so carefully designed and executed that it may convince some of the skeptics of the importance of the mind-body connection.

Many people with TMS report a history of hypertension, suggesting that the same emotional states may bring on either of these. Just a few weeks ago, a patient called and reported that her back pain was gone but that she had now developed hypertension—a clear example of equivalency.

By contrast, it is rare for a TMS patient to report a history of *coronary artery disease* or subsequently to develop it. I can document the former, but I do not have statistics to support the latter; it is a clinical impression.

Almost everyone has heard of the so-called Type A behavior pattern and of the susceptibility of Type A people to coronary artery disease, described by Dr. Meyer Friedman and Dr. Ray Rosenman in their 1974 book, *Type A Behavior and Your Heart.*

Type A people were described as extremely ambitious, aggressive, loving competition, obsessively hard workers, often putting themselves under great time pressure, having much need for recognition, and very hostile. Because of their tendency to be compulsive, perfectionistic, and very responsible and conscientious, people with TMS often describe themselves as Type A. They are, in fact, different in some important respects. Many TMS patients are the antithesis of hostile; they often have a strong need to be good, nice, pleasant, accommodating, and helpful. Though they may be ambitious and often very accomplished, they do not necessarily pursue their goals with the intensity that seems to be characteristic of the Type A person.

After the publication of *Type A Behavior and Your Heart,* a great deal of research was done in an attempt to clarify the relative importance of the various Type A traits. It has been suggested that of all those listed above, hostility may be the only one that predisposes someone to coronary artery disease.

To someone who is aware of being angry a lot, this can be disturbing, whether or not he or she has TMS. It is of great interest to me because of the increasing evidence that repressed anger is important in the psychological dynamics of TMS. But then how does one reconcile those facts with the clear statistical evidence in the TMS population that coronary artery disease is very rare?

It is apparent that a great deal more research and thinking is needed to unravel this mystery. It is dangerous to focus on a trait like hostility without knowing a great deal more than we do about the psychodynamics of anger or about the myriad details of people's personalities. The man who swears at taxi drivers as he drives down the street may be displacing his anger at his boss this way, for it is far better than losing his job. Or it may be much more complicated than that.

The problem with the behavioral research typified here is that it is unidimensional. It draws conclusions based upon oversimplified models of human behavior. This is one of the weaknesses of contemporary research in this area. In an attempt to produce statistically valid conclusions, it must use criteria that are measurable, and while this is appropriate, it places a great burden on the investigator to be absolutely sure that he knows what he is measuring. This is perfectly illustrated by the history of Type A behavior research.

To make matters worse for the poor person who sees himself angry a lot of the time, it is suggested *that he stop doing it!* This makes him downright desperate. He has been told that this kind of behavior is liable to give him a heart attack and to avoid it he had better stop being who he is.

I would not presume to advise anyone who believes that he or she is a Type A person. I tell my TMS patients that, statistically, they appear not to be prone to coronary artery disease. If they are aware of being angry a lot of the time, they are already ahead of the game, because they are aware. If they are really concerned about this tendency, I am prepared to introduce them to a psychotherapist who will help them to learn more about why they behave as they do. In my experience, awareness is very good medicine.

The wonderful thing about the whole Type A story is that it has convinced some of the medical community that what is going on in the mind may be of great importance to what's happening in the body—at least as far as coronary artery disease is concerned.

Hardening of the arteries, arteriosclerosis, the deposition of arteriosclerotic plaques—these all mean the same thing. Since what narrows the coronary arteries are arteriosclerotic plaques and a relationship has been established between emotions and coronary artery disease, one is tempted to theorize about hardening of the arteries in general. *Arteriosclerosis* refers to the laying down of these crusty plaques on the inside of blood vessels that may retard the flow of blood or be the basis of blood clots that then occlude the artery. In light of the work of Dr. Friedman and Dr. Rosenman, it is hard to escape the conclusion that emotions may play a role in hardening of the arteries wherever it occurs, though it is clear that genetics (it pays to pick the right parents), blood pressure, diet, weight, and exercise all play important roles.

An important report was published in the prestigious British journal *Lancet* in July 1990 (Vol. 336, pp. 129–33). A large team headed by Dr. Dean Ornish of the University of California San Francisco School of Medicine did a randomized, controlled study in which they demonstrated that lifestyle changes (practiced for a year) could actually reverse the process of atherosclerosis (arteriosclerosis, hardening) in coronary arteries. The patients in the experimental group were put on a low-fat, low-cholesterol vegetarian diet; participated in stress-management activities like meditation, relaxation, imagery, breathing techniques, and stretching exercises; and did moderate aerobic exercise regularly. In addition, there were twice-weekly group discussions to provide social support and reinforce adherence to the lifestyle change program. The control (nonexperimental) group of patients showed an increase in coronary atherosclerosis. With the decrease in blockage of the coronary arteries, experimental patients also experienced a reduction in the frequency, duration, and severity of angina (chest pain) while the control group had an increase in angina over the one-year period.

This obviously important report shows what has long been suspected: that it is not just diet, exercise, and other purely physical factors that determine whether or not there will be hardening of the arteries but psychosocial factors as well. I predict that further experimentation will identify the person's emotional state as being the most important variable and that intensive psychotherapy alone will demonstrate a similar reversal of atherosclerosis.

Heart palpitation to the layman usually means a very rapid heart rate. The medical term for this is *tachycardia,* with rates from 130 to 200 beats a minute. The most common form of this is paroxysmal auricular tachycardia (PAT), and, in my experience, it is usually induced by emotional factors. Regardless of that, it should always be treated by one's family doctor, internist, or cardiologist. Ideally, the emotional reason for the attack should be explored.

Irregularity of heart rhythm may also be referred to as *palpitation.* I have experienced these intermittently all my life, and, again, they are clearly the result of emotional things. They, too, should be investigated and managed by your doctor to be sure they are not the result of a cardiac abnormality. It is generally accepted that these conditions are mediated through the autonomic nervous system.

Finally, a disorder known as *mitral valve prolapse* is a very common abnormality of one of the leaflets of a heart valve. The leaflet becomes "floppy" and does not perform normally, so that a murmur can often be heard. It sounds scary but is very common, occurs more often in women than in men, and seems not to be associated with functional disability. I have had it for years and continue to be very active, and I perform vigorous aerobic activity on a regular basis.

What is intriguing about it is that some doctors think it is psychogenic—that is, anxiety induced. And there is considerable evidence in the medical literature that it is related to abnormal autonomic activity (editorial in the *Lancet*, October 3, 1987, titled, "Autonomic Function in Mitral Valve Prolapse").

Recently an article appeared in the July 1989 issue of *Archives of Physical Medicine and Rehabilitation* (Vol. 90, pp. 541–43) reporting a study in which 75 percent of a group of patients with fibromyalgia were found to have mitral valve prolapse, a higher incidence of this disorder than in the general population. As I have stated, I believe fibromyalgia to be one of the forms of TMS.

Since TMS and mitral valve prolapse are both induced by abnormal autonomic activity and TMS is clearly the result of emotional factors, it is tempting to include mitral valve prolapse in that list of physical disorders that have their genesis in the realm of the emotions. Using myself as an example, I have experienced TMS, gastrointestinal symptoms, migraine headache, hay fever, dermatologic conditions, and mitral valve prolapse, and so have a large number of my TMS patients, suggesting that the same thing is at the root of all of them—repressed, undesirable emotions.

Let me repeat a very important point: The idea that emotions can stimulate physiologic change is impossible for most physicians to accept, and they are, therefore, cut off from the possibility of understanding a large number of ills that now plague human beings. TMS and mitral valve prolapse surely fall into that group.

In summary, five cardiovascular disorders probably related to the emotions have been briefly described. It is of great interest that three of the five, hypertension, palpitations, and mitral valve prolapse, are mediated through the autonomic nervous system.

THE MIND AND THE IMMUNE SYSTEM

Contemplation of the complexity of animal biology is awe inspiring and overwhelming. It is impossible to imagine how something as complicated as we are came to be. Little wonder that it took millions of years to evolve.

The immune system is a marvel of complexity and efficiency. It is designed to protect us from foreign invaders of all kinds, the most important of which are infectious agents, and from dangerous enemies that are generated within, like cancer. It is composed of a variety of defense strategies: It can generate chemicals to kill invaders; it can mobilize armies of cells to swallow them up; and it has an elaborate system whereby it can recognize thousands of substances that are foreign to our bodies and then neutralize them.

For years it was thought by immunologists to be an autonomous system, though there were disconcerting stories about patients along the way that suggested that the mind might have something to do with the way it worked. For the most part, these stories were discounted by the experts, but now there is concrete evidence that cannot be ignored that the brain is involved in the system.

Robert Ader, a research psychologist at the University of Rochester, was engaged in an experiment in which he was trying to condition rats to dislike saccharin-sweetened water. This was similar to the classic experiment of Pavlov in which he conditioned dogs to salivate at the sound of a bell. In order to develop an aversion to the saccharin, Dr. Ader injected the rats with a chemical that made them nauseated so that they associated the sweet water with nausea. What he didn't realize until later was that the chemical he injected, cyclophosphamide, also suppressed the rats' immune systems, so that they were dying mysteriously. But the striking thing was that now all he had to do was feed the rats saccharin-sweetened water and their immune systems would be suppressed, even though they had not been injected with the chemical, because they had learned (been conditioned) to associate the sweet water with the nausea-producing chemical. Now, simply feeding saccharin could produce suppression of the immune system. This was a landmark discovery, for it demonstrated that a brain phenomenon, in this case aversion to a taste, could control the immune system.

It is no wonder, then, that people with TMS can experience pain under the weirdest of circumstances, like when they are lying quietly on their stomachs. They have been told that lying on the stomach is bad for the back, so they become conditioned to have an aversion to that posture and, naturally, will then experience pain. As stated earlier, the brain can influence any organ or system in the body. In the case of Dr. Ader's rats, it was the immune system; with TMS, it is the autonomic system.

Something else observed by Dr. Ader and his co-workers was that rats who had autoimmune diseases improved during such experiments. This is because this group of disorders results when the immune system turns on the body and produces substances that are harmful to some of the body's own tissues (rheumatoid arthritis, diabetes, lupus erythematosus, and multiple sclerosis are examples of such diseases). That means that anything that suppresses the immune system will allow those disorders to improve, which is what happened when autoimmune-diseased rats were fed saccharin water.

The implications of this for human health and illness are enormous, since autoimmune disorders are among the most problematic and poorly understood of all categories of disease. These experiments suggest that the brain might play a role in the treatment of these conditions. It further suggests to me that emotions may play a role in their *cause*.

In his well-known book *The Anatomy of an Illness,* Norman Cousins described how he overcame one of these autoimmune disorders, ankylosing spondylitis (a form of rheumatoid arthritis), by recognizing that it was emotionally induced and introducing a kind of humor therapy plus vitamin C. Based on my experience with TMS, I am inclined to think that it was his recognition of the role of the emotions in causing the illness that produced the cure. It is possible that, just as in TMS, the illness serves to draw attention away from the realm of the emotions and that when the person recognizes that this is what is going on, and attention is focused on the emotions, the illness loses its purpose and ceases.

Those of us who believe that the immune system is heavily influenced by the emotions are in debt to Dr. Ader for having shown in the laboratory that this is a reality. He is not alone; other laboratory scientists have demonstrated equally dramatic connections between mind and body.

One report that particularly impressed me appeared in the prestigious journal *Science* in April 1982 by authors Visintainer, Volpicelli, and Seligman. They described a group of rats, all suffering from the same cancer, that were exposed to annoying electric shock under two different experimental conditions; one group could escape from it, and the other had to take it until it stopped. Both groups got exactly the same dose of shock; the ability to escape from it was the only difference between the two groups. According to the authors, "Rats receiving inescapable shock were only half as likely to reject the tumor and twice as likely to die as rats receiving escapable shock or no shock. Only 27 percent of the rats given inescapable shock rejected the tumor, compared to 63 percent of the rats given escapable shock and 54 percent of the rats given no shock."

The clear implication of the study was that the immune systems of the rats that were more emotionally stressed were less efficient, since it is the effectiveness of the immune system that determines whether a cancer will be thrown off or not. If this is the case with rats, imagine how much more important the emotions must be in humans.

CANCER AND THE IMMUNE SYSTEM

Since the subject of the emotions and cancer has been introduced, let's pursue it further. Though it is not yet under intensive research by mainstream medicine, there have been many observations through the years that psychological and social factors may play a role in the cause and cure of cancer.

One of these was reported by Kenneth Pelletier, a member of the faculty of the School of Medicine, University of California, at the time. He was interested in "miracle cancer cures" that had occurred in seven people in the San Francisco area and wondered if they had anything in common. He found, in fact, that all seven people became more outgoing, more community oriented, interested in things outside of themselves; they all tried to change their lives so that there was more time for pleasurable activities; all seven became religious, in different ways, but all looked to something bigger than themselves; each spent a period of time each day meditating, sitting quietly, and contemplating or praying; they all started a physical exercise program, and they all changed their diets to include less red meat and more vegetables. It certainly looks as though social and emotional factors played a role in these "miracle cures."

Pelletier is the author of a well-known book about the mind-body connection, *Mind as Healer, Mind as Slayer* (New York: Delacorte, 1977).

For those interested, there is a book by O. Carl Simonton, Stephanie Matthews-Simonton, and James Creighton titled *Getting Well Again* (New York: J. P. Tarcher, 1978) that describes the Simontons' therapeutic technique for treating cancer. Theirs is a psychological approach to the problem in which they seek to understand their patients and find ways of changing attitudes and concepts, since they believe these are important to the eventual outcome.

A very popular recent book on the subject is *Love, Medicine, and Miracles* by the Yale surgeon Bernie Siegel (New York: Harper & Row, 1986). Dr. Siegel began his career as a surgeon, became aware of the social and psychological dimensions of cancer, and began to work with patients accordingly. His book is highly inspirational and, because of its popularity, has introduced many people to the idea that the mind can be mobilized to combat cancer.

There may be some cause for concern about the nature of Dr. Siegel's work, however, because of its lack of psychological and physiologic specificity. He does not present a theoretical model of how emotions play a role in the cause and cure of cancer and where his work fits into that model. Lacking that, it is unlikely that his work will have much impact on the traditional medical research community.

This is a pity, for there is a great need for more precise definition of *what* social and psychological factors are contributing to *what* illnesses and how. Acknowledging the important role of the emotions in health and illness, medicine must reexamine its concepts of disease causation. The attempt to bridge that mysterious gap between emotion and physiology will require the best minds in experimental medicine and the kind of interest and commitment that medicine now accords to such things as genetic research or the chemotherapy of cancer.

But we won't get those people and that kind of commitment if we put "the power of love" into a medical context without carefully studying its specific psychological and physiologic effects. If that isn't done, how do we distinguish between Bernie Siegel, Norman Vincent Peale, and Mary Baker Eddy?

These considerations aside, doctors like Siegel, Simonton, Pelletier, and Locke (and a number of others I have not mentioned) are pioneers, and what they have to teach is of enormous importance to the future of medicine.

THE IMMUNE SYSTEM AND INFECTIOUS DISEASES

Here again, there is a long history of awareness that the emotions have something to do with our susceptibility to or ability to fight off infection, but none of it is generally accepted by medical doctors and rarely applied in everyday practice. Frequent colds and genitourinary infections are among the most common, but it is likely that psychological factors play a role in all infectious processes.

As with cancer, it is the efficiency of the immune system to do its job of eradicating the infectious agent that is at issue. Stressful emotions can reduce that effectiveness and allow the infection to flourish, but there is ample anecdotal evidence that people have the capacity to enhance immunologic efficiency by improving their emotional states or employing other techniques, as the following story illustrates.

The cover article of the *Washington Post Health Journal* for January 1985 was a piece written by Sally Squires titled "The Mind Fights Back." In it she described a study carried out by a team of immunologists and psychiatrists at the University of Arkansas Medical Sciences in which a woman described as a "dedicated meditator" who was particularly attuned to her body's responses was chosen to participate in this interesting experiment.

Chicken pox virus was injected into her forearm. Having been previously exposed to the virus, she developed the usual positive immune reaction, a bump about one-half inch in diameter, which then disappeared in a few days. To confirm that an immune reaction was going on, a blood test was done that demonstrated that her white blood cells were actively fighting the infection. After repeating the procedure twice with the same reaction, she was instructed to try to stop the body's normal reaction, which she did in her daily meditation, and for three weeks in a row the bump got smaller and smaller. Then she was asked to stop interfering with the normal immune reaction, and with the last three injections of the virus, she got the usual bump again.

Here was a clear demonstration of how the mind can alter a bodily reaction if it is taught how to do it. The doctors involved in the study were so impressed with the results that they repeated the entire experiment nine months later and got the same results.

Conventional medical research can hardly find fault with this experiment. It was a striking demonstration of the so-called power of the mind, in this case over the working of the immune system.

The treatment of TMS describes a similar phenomenon, in which acquired knowledge has the ability to interfere with an undesirable physical reaction, the pain of TMS.

THE OVERACTIVE
IMMUNE SYSTEM—ALLERGY

Though the idea is controversial, it is my view, based on experience with patients who have had both TMS and allergic rhinitis (hay fever), that some of the common allergies of adult life are equivalents of TMS—that is, they are brought on by emotional factors. People invariably say when this is discussed, "Oh, but hay fever is caused by things like pollens, dust, and molds; how can you say it's due to tension?" If ten people are standing in a field of grass pollen, not all of them will begin to sneeze, only the allergic ones. What is the difference between the nonallergic and the allergic people? The immune systems of the latter have become overactive under the influence of tension, the repressed feelings we have been talking about. This has been demonstrated, not occasionally, but repeatedly in TMS patients who have been told in the course of their learning experience that hay fever is a TMS equivalent and can be eliminated in the same way that TMS can. And they do it.

Mr. G. reported at one of the small group meetings that he has suffered from fall hay fever for seventeen years— but not this year! He took to heart what he had heard and, miracle, experienced no hay fever that season.

For years I have been allergic to whatever it is that cats exude (we used to call it *dander,* but now we're told it may be something in their saliva that dries on their meticulously licked fur and then floats into the air). If I walk into a house and don't know that a cat lives there, my eyes begin to itch. I usually start rubbing them without thinking. Then kitty walks into the room and I say, "Ah—now I know the reason for the itchy eyes," and they stop itching. That happens because I know that allergic rhinitis and conjunctivitis are two of my mind's tension repertoire, and as stated in chapter 4 on treatment, to recognize these conditions for what they are is to invalidate them—and symptoms then cease.

Most of the medical community rejects the idea that emotions have anything to do with allergy. These two examples can't be explained in any other way. They show that something is at work besides an autonomous immune system reacting to inhaled substances; how could one get the symptoms to stop simply by thinking? Clearly, the same mental-emotional dynamics are at work here as those described in the treatment chapter.

I do not have evidence that this "knowledge therapy" will work with any of the other common allergies, and so I will say nothing about them, except if I had one of them, I would certainly zero in on emotional factors in my life.

Incidentally, acknowledging the role of emotions does not preclude the use of conventional medical treatment.

MIND AND THE
GASTROINTESTINAL SYSTEM

This is the one area where there is a tradition for recognizing the role of emotional factors, among physicians and laymen alike. However, while most people would still say that ulcers are caused by tension, doctors are trying very hard to prove that they are not. Peruse any medical journal specializing in disorders of the gastrointestinal system (there is one with the colorful name *Gut*) and you will find many articles suggesting a variety of purely "physical" causes, with nary a mention of emotions. This is in keeping with the trend already mentioned to focus more and more on the physics and chemistry of illness.

In the course of my work with TMS over seventeen years, I have seen a consistent correlation with gastrointestinal (GI) conditions. Patients will often have a history of heartburn, hiatus hernia (which seems to be part of the ulcer syndrome), peptic ulcer, irritable bowel syndrome, spastic colon, constipation, or "gas," to name the most common. These are things they have usually had prior to their pain problems.

As with TMS, they are the result of what I have called abnormal autonomic function, in turn stimulated, in my view, by the same emotional factors that are responsible for TMS. They are less common now than they were thirty or forty years ago, but that is because TMS has become the preferred physical defense against anxiety and anger. Another likely reason is the advent of excellent antiulcer medications. Since the drugs can eliminate the symptoms, there is no longer anything to capture the person's attention, which is the purpose of a psychophysiologic process—so the brain chooses something else, like TMS. This decline in incidence has been documented in medical literature.

The most striking evidence that these GI conditions are emotion related and can be attacked in the same way as TMS is the story of the man who accompanied his wife to the lectures and experienced relief of his lifelong stomach symptoms on learning how the mind affects the body (described earlier in this chapter).

MIND AND HEADACHE

Persistent or recurrent headache should always be investigated by one's regular physician. Though rare, it may be a sign of something serious like a tumor.

I don't intend an exhaustive review of the subject of headache here but simply will say that in my experience, the majority of headache is of the tension variety, which makes it a close relative of TMS. I suspect the mechanism is exactly the same, with constriction of small blood vessels feeding scalp muscles. As with TMS, the basic cause is tension, as we have defined it, and there is a wide variety of patterns and severity.

Those that involve the back of the head are clearly related to the posterior neck muscles that are part of TMS. Some patients report pain all over the head; others have it in the frontal region. A common complaint is of severe pain "behind the eyes." When they are unilateral (involving one side only), severe, and are accompanied by nausea, people are inclined to call them migraines. Tension headache can be as disabling as the worst neck, shoulder, or back pain.

Migraine headache appears to have the same underlying psychological cause as tension headache but has a different physiology. I had migraines for a number of years and can speak with the authority of the sufferer. What distinguishes them from tension headache is some sort of neurological phenomenon, usually visual, preceding the onset of the headache. I had a jagged, curved line that occupied varying parts of my visual field. It looked like cracked glass, and it "scintillated"—that is, it flashed on and off very rapidly. For some reason they are called "lights." They usually started with a small dot that obscured a part of the visual field and over a period of minutes developed into the full-blown pattern described above. The phenomenon lasted about fifteen minutes, gradually faded out, and was then followed by the headache, which could go on to become very severe.

What is a little scary about migraine is that it has been well established that it is due to constriction of a blood vessel within the substance of the brain. Once I had an episode during which my speech was incoherent for about an hour, something called *aphasia*, the result of the temporary constriction of a vital artery in the speech area of the brain.

But the good news about migraine is that it, too, is an equivalent of TMS and can be stopped in precisely the same manner, at least in my experience. It happened to me years before I knew anything about TMS. I was a young family practitioner, having an occasional migraine, when I had a conversation with one of the older physicians in the community who said that he had read somewhere that migraines might be due to repressed anger. The next time I got the "lights," which meant I had about fifteen minutes to think, I tried to figure out what I might be angry about but came up with a blank. However, to my amazement, I did not get the headache—and I have never had another one to this day, though I continue to get the "lights" a few times a year.

In retrospect, I know very well why I was getting migraines way back then and what I was repressing. Now when I get the warning signal, I can usually figure out what I am angry about and am constantly struck by the fact that no matter how many times I recognize that I have repressed anger, I will do it again and again, for it is apparently part of my nature, the way I developed psychologically, to do this. But see how powerful knowledge can be. By recognizing what I was doing, I was able to stop a very nasty physical reaction. Just as with TMS.

MIND AND THE SKIN:
ACNE AND WARTS

There appears to be a close connection between these skin disorders and the emotions. As with virtually all of these mind-body processes, there is no laboratory proof of the causative role of emotions, but there is certainly a mountain of clinical evidence. Acne is one of the common "other things" that people with TMS have had or continue to have even while they're having back trouble.

And then there's the story of the man who developed an itchy rash under his wedding band that disappeared as soon as he separated from his wife. Other gold rings did not produce a similar rash.

It has been suggested that other skin disorders like eczema and psoriasis are related to the emotions. I am inclined to agree but have no evidence one way or the other.

THE WITCH DOCTOR

Evidences of the power of the mind are all around us. The placebo reaction is ubiquitous. Most practitioners owe some of their success to this phenomenon, and some would have no success at all were it not for the placebo effect.

Years ago I found a wonderful example of mind-body interaction in an article by Louis C. Whiton in the August–September 1971 issue of *Natural History* magazine titled "Under the Power of the Gran Gadu" (Vol. 80, No. 7). Dr. Whiton had been conducting anthropological studies in Surinam, South America, for years and was particularly interested in the ceremonies, rituals, and cures of tribal witch doctors from a group of jungle people known as Bush Negroes. He had been suffering for two years from a painful condition of the right hip attributed to trochanteric bursitis (see page 137). It had been resistant to all treatment. Accompanied by his personal physician, five friends, and the editor of a Surinamese newspaper, he traveled forty miles into the forest out of Paramaribo to be treated by a highly reputed witch doctor named Raineh. There was a picture of Raineh in Dr. Whiton's article, and he was a very impressive-looking man.

Described in great detail by Dr. Whiton, the ceremony began at midnight and went on for four and a half hours. There were many steps: The patient had to be protected from evil spirits, his soul had to be interrogated about his past life, beneficent local gods were attracted, it was necessary to "pull the witch" out of the patient's body and transfer it to that of the witch doctor. It was at that point that Dr. Whiton arose from the ground and found that his pain was gone. The ceremony went on to transfer the "witch" from the body of the doctor to that of a chicken and concluded with incantations and other procedures to prevent the "evil" from reentering the patient's body.

Dr. Whiton was no doubt disposed to having a successful therapeutic experience, for he had confidence in the power of the mind to heal the body. Nevertheless, that predisposition was of no value to him here in the United States. He needed a healer of power and stature—and he found him in the forest of Surinam.

I do not subscribe to placebo cures, for, as I have said elsewhere, they are usually temporary. But this story is told because it is another example of what the mind can do.

DR. H. K. BEECHER

Dr. H. K. Beecher is the name of one of the first serious students of pain in the United States. In 1946, he published an article in the *Annals of Surgery* titled "Pain in Men Wounded in Battle" (Vol. 123, p. 96). For years it was widely quoted because of its most interesting observation. But now Dr. Beecher is passing into obscurity, for what he had to say is no longer acceptable to students of pain.

Dr. Beecher questioned 215 seriously wounded soldiers at various locations in the European theater during World War II shortly after they had been wounded and found that 75 percent of them had so little pain that they had no need for morphine. Reflecting that strong emotion can block pain, Dr. Beecher went on to speculate: "In this connection it is important to consider the position of the soldier: His wound suddenly releases him from an exceedingly dangerous environment, one filled with fatigue, discomfort, anxiety, fear and real danger of death, and gives him a ticket to the safety of the hospital. His troubles are over, or he thinks they are."

This observation is reinforced by a report of the United States surgeon general during World War II, noted in Martin Gilbert's book *The Second World War: A Complete History* (New York: Henry Holt, 1989), that in order to avoid psychiatric breakdown, infantrymen had to be relieved of duty every so often. The report said, "A wound or injury is regarded not as a misfortune, but a blessing."

Here is yet another way in which the mind can modify or eliminate pain. Good spirits, a joyful attitude, a positive emotional state clearly have the ability to block or prevent pain. Just how this works one cannot know at this time.

But we do know in part how the therapeutic process in TMS works. The knowledge of what the brain is about renders the process purposeless, the abnormal autonomic stimuli cease, and so does the pain. What we have yet to discover, and it is probably beyond our mental horizons to do so at this time, is how emotional phenomena can stimulate physiologic ones. That they do is unquestionable, but for the time being, we may have to be content with Benjamin Franklin's observation: "Nor is it of much Importance to us to know the Manner in which Nature executes her Laws: tis enough to know the Laws themselves."

APPENDIX

Letters from Patients

Many patients have written to me, relating their experiences with TMS and the results they achieved with my book.

I'll let them speak for themselves. . . .

Dear Dr. Sarno:

This letter is a follow-up to my letter written to you around the beginning of July 1987. . . . I am happy to report that my back problem *was* TMS and I have been able to get rid of the pain to a degree of about 95 percent. Once in a great while I notice some pain, but after getting the causes of stress out of my mind (not necessarily out of my life!) I made major progress. My worst problem had been the inability to sit, and since I do office work it was very difficult. I used a chair for months that is designed to put most of the weight on the knees, but I can now sit in regular chairs for lengthy periods of time and don't even *think* about my back!

Dear Dr. Sarno:

Your letter . . . has finally reached me . . . where I have been for the past three weeks caring for my sick mother. This has certainly been a test of whether my back would begin to hurt again! . . . I know my back wouldn't even hurt except for the fatigue of caring for an elderly person constantly, making the decision to put her in a "personal care residence" . . . where my brother lives and then going to her home and spending a week packing everything and putting the house up for sale. Certainly a cause for stress!

Anyway, the good news is I have *not* allowed this situation to stress me out. . . . I know after I return home . . . and get a few days of rest I'll be fine.

. . . I think your TMS theory is accurate and I want as many people as possible to benefit from your research. . . .

Dr. Sarno:

. . . My back pain started in my lower back when I was in my mid-twenties (I am now thirty-four). By the time I turned thirty, my pain had spread throughout my back, neck and shoulders. The pain was chronic, and often debilitating. After useless sessions with my family practice doctor, and then with a neurologist, I turned to chiropractic care on a friend's recommendation. After two and a half years of "adjustments" one to three times a week, my pain was reduced and under control, but not permanently cured. As a naval officer, I have overseas duty or possibly sea duty in the not so distant future, and I knew that my dependence on chiropractic care would have to end if I wanted to continue my naval career. It was in the midst of struggling with this dilemma that a friend of a relative referred me to your work. . . .

. . . I realized that your stereotype of a TMS sufferer described me to a tee. Moreover, your thorough physiological explanation of TMS made sense to me as nothing I heard (from doctors) or read beforehand. What a relief to *finally* find someone who not only understood what I had been experiencing, but offered hope as well based on sound medical reasoning and experience! I immediately accepted TMS as my diagnosis. (My acceptance was probably hastened by the knowledge that a veteran Navy back specialist had recently conducted a detailed examination of a complete set of back and neck X-rays, and concluded that I had no spinal misalignment, no abnormal discs and no signs of arthritis.) After two more readings of your book, and about two months' time, my back and neck pain had essentially disappeared. A couple of weeks later the pain returned, but I simply refocused my thoughts on the TMS diagnosis, and the pain disappeared once again after about a week. Since that time, I have experienced a couple of other relapses, but the same type of knowledge therapy quickly defuses them, and the relapses are becoming progressively shorter in duration.

. . . I consider my TMS under control. I know that it will probably never go away completely, but I feel confident that I can control it without depending on a chiropractor or medical doctor or anyone else. I am enjoying my wife and small children once again, my naval career is back on track, and I have great hope for the future. . . .

Dear Dr. Sarno:

. . . In 1970 I was diagnosed as having a slipped disc. I managed pretty well until 1979 when I had another bad bout. A second doctor (I saw four that year—two said slipped disc, two said not) told me I had two vertebrae too close together and this caused a muscular imbalance. I did exercises religiously twice a day (thereafter until this spring). They got me out of bed (I spent a lot of 1979 in bed) but I was never as good. Then in 1986 I got worse. The insides of my upper legs were trembly and ached a lot. I was getting scared. I feared back surgery, because the results are so mixed with people.

After reading your book, I began ignoring the pain and, more crucially, quit fearing the pain and now I do what I want. I still have some discomfort but I keep going and it dissipates.

This is a wonderful book. The syndrome you can get into, the vicious circle of pain, bed rest, more pain, fear, fear, fear. It hems you in and is so depressing. I waited a few months to see if this was really going to work over the long haul. It's going to, so I'm writing to say: Thank you.

Dear Dr. Sarno:

. . . It is now approximately sixteen months since I recovered from what was diagnosed as a herniated L-5 disc with sciatic nerve pain. I had seen two well-respected orthopedists associated with [a noted] Medical School and a chiropractor before reading your book, all of whom assured me that my CT scan findings and clinical symptoms made my diagnosis certain. I was ordered to remain in bed for several weeks, given anti-inflammatory medications, and told to hope for uncertain recovery.

For almost four months I lived with considerable pain and terrible limitations of my mobility. I work as a clinical psychologist and had to lie down to see patients. Driving was terribly painful, and I felt that I could only walk short distances. My previously active, athletic lifestyle was becoming a memory. As my incapacitation dragged on, I worried about needing surgery, the outcome of which was uncertain.

Upon initial reading of your book, I was skeptical, though I could not help but become excited. Despite my training as a psychologist, I had accepted the mechanical explanations of disc injury offered by the orthopedic doctors without question. I had noticed that my pain was worse when I was tense, but this didn't alter my view of my "injury." Your book offered an alternate, scientifically plausible explanation for me to consider.

It was clear to me that I thought about little but my back and leg pain, and I was extremely fearful about my every movement. The image of further injuring my spine was always with me. As I read your book, it occurred to me that my first symptoms had occurred around the time of an emotionally stressful event. I had once before suffered from gastrointestinal problems during a stressful time, so that the thought that my back problem might have started as a somatization disorder made some sense to me.

On the advice of a friend who had also been "cured" by your book, I tried becoming more active, despite my pain. While my first forays into increased activity were terrifying, I soon realized that they didn't make my pain worse. I also noticed that the pain moved from one leg to another, despite my CT scan showing a protrusion on only the right side. This observation was very encouraging. I recall the moment when, after walking around the block and noticing pain in my left as well as right leg, I started laughing with joy. You were right! This whole ordeal was muscle tension—my life wasn't really ruined!

Within two weeks after this realization, I had my life back. I began taking long walks and sitting normally. The pain was diminishing gradually. I noticed that when someone mentioned the word *disc* in a conversation, my pain increased. I had to reread your book several times to keep my confidence going, and after each reading, my pain lessened. I avoided contact with my orthopedist and people who believed that they have structural back problems, because I was still too tentative in my new understanding and the cycle of fear-pain-fear-pain was readily reactivated by thinking that you might be wrong.

When I began to recover, I saw a physical therapist who thought that your ideas were plausible and helped me to increase my range of motion and rebuild my muscle strength. In retrospect, she was most helpful in making me feel safe about moving again.

During the past year I have been unrestricted in my physical activities. I have done many things which should be terrible for a herniated L-5 disc and sciatic pain, such as fly to Thailand (twenty-six hours of airplane sitting), build a room in the basement, ski, hike, lift babies and hike with a backpack. I rarely feel sciatic nerve pain, and when I do it is mild. I no longer think about my back;

instead I think about what may be making me feel anxious or tense. I experience my sciatic nerve as a benign barometer of anxiety.

I know . . . that you have heard many stories such as mine. I hope that this letter can be of use to others who are suffering from what for me was an iatrogenic disorder caused by my orthopedist's misunderstanding of what began as a harmless somatization problem. . . .

Dear Dr. Sarno:

I am delighted to offer my comments concerning your book and its effect on me.

In the summer of 1987 while playing tennis, I suffered a sudden, incapacitating "event" in my back. I had had some minor back problems as a teenager but had been symptom free for over twenty years. (I am forty-one years old now.) I managed to get to work but when my boss, who had (and still has) back problems which eventually led to surgery, saw me he ordered me home and to a doctor immediately.

At the doctor's office, the orthopedist lugged out the model of a spinal column showing me how nerves can get wedged between bone and cartilage and create the terrible spasm I was experiencing. His advice was to get into bed for two weeks and to certainly not go on the weeklong bicycle trip I had planned for ten days hence. I immediately broke out in a cold sweat over the prospect of missing two weeks of work and the apparent seriousness of my malady based on that long convalescence.

Well, I actually stayed in bed for five days and then returned to work, still in pain. Unable to sit up for extended periods of time, I spent a few hours a day on the floor in my office with my telephone by my side. Then, armed with Motrin and Robaxin that the doctor described, I went on the bike trip. Strangely, I actually found that my back was feeling better as the week wore on, despite the fact that I was propped up on a bicycle seat for five hours a day (ah ha, clue # 1).

For the next ten months I had a few other less severe incidents. Each time I had one of these occurrences, I put away my running shoes and tennis gear and waited for the pain to subside (all the while visualizing my spinal cord being sawed in half by a disc pressing on the vertebrae). Then in the spring of 1988, coincident with a particularly stressful situation in my personal life, I suffered an attack that persisted for weeks. At about the same time, a friend . . . who had had chronic back problems for years, told me about you. I was dubious—to say the least. . . .

I guess you could say that the two round-trip commutes . . . to New York that it took me to read the book changed my life. It's embarrassing to think that I am so typical but on the other hand it was reassuring to learn how normal I am. The book made perfectly clear to me that although the back spasms were indeed real, they were a function of muscles deprived of sufficient blood flow. . . .

While I feel society may have unrealistic and unfair expectations about the power of self-healing (such as attaching implicit blame on cancer victims for their inability to conquer their disease), I am now absolutely convinced that so much of our well-being is within the grasp of each of us. Your book has simply showed me the direction to go when a problem arises.

Dear Dr. Sarno:

Your book was literally a relief. The attached letter to my doctor perhaps best sums up my situation. . . .

I hope my written gratitude accurately reflects the relief your book has given to me and my wife. Thank you.

Dear Doctor:

I am writing to tell you how I progressed since I last saw you in November. When we last spoke, you had reviewed the results of an MRI I had taken. At that time I was close to acquiescing to your recommendation for surgery; I had not improved after extended bed rest and subsequently an MRI appeared to show a herniated disc.

After I saw you I tried a chiropractor, but he was no help. The pain in my leg would get better at times and worse at others; there were no definitive patterns. Then at Christmastime I canceled all vacation plans and decided to spend three weeks on my back. But after one week I was in more pain than ever. Frankly, I was terribly worried. I had almost resigned myself to adjusting to a restricted lifestyle. That is until a family member sent me a book on back pain which I feel you should know about.

The book was spectacular because it attributed my back pain, after a thorough description of the pain and likeness, to muscle spasm brought on by tension. The cure: to get out of bed and resume life as normal—get the blood circulating to cramped muscles, and relax!

APPENDIX

The first thing I did after reading the book—and mind you I was in unbearable pain—was get in the car, ditch the back rest and drive four hours straight. When I finally parked the car I had no pain. The following three or four days, I sat almost the entire day without a break, and I took brisk walks on a sandy beach. The pain increasingly disappeared. A week and a half later, I played racquetball for an hour and a half and won all three games—no pain whatsoever.

The muscle spasm diagnosis made sense because no particular incident brought on the pain, rather it sprang up when I quit my job to enter graduate school without having first been admitted. I was trying to change my career field and I had either to jump then or perhaps never at all. At that time you would not have been pulling my leg to have told me I was "stressed out."

My main objective in writing this account is to thank you for your time and patience and, most importantly, to help others. . . .

Dear Dr. Sarno:

I want to thank you for how much you have helped my health and therefore the quality of my life. . . .

I had been suffering from severe back pain (both upper and lower, including sciatic) for seven years at the time I called you. I also had regular severe intestinal cramps; intense sharp pains in my chest; pain in my knees, ankles, elbows, wrists, knuckles and one shoulder.

All this pain, especially the back pain, severely limited

my ability to work and play. I could not sweep the floor, do dishes, pick up babies (or anything over about three pounds, for that matter), join in sports, etc. Even brushing my hair hurt.

I had been a very strong, active person with a great need to exert myself physically—which I (and everyone else) blamed as the cause of my back problems.

On the first visit to my doctor, I was told to back off as much activity as possible, to do nothing that hurt, and that probably a lot of things would hurt.

I followed that advice. Over the next seven years, I became an "expert" on the supposed causes and cures of back pain, but to no avail. I had fourteen sessions of acupuncture, seventeen chiropractic sessions, seventeen "body balancing" sessions, thirteen rolfing sessions, several physical therapy sessions, used a "neuro-block TENS unit," attended "bad-back exercise class," joined a health spa—went swimming and used a Jacuzzi and sauna, received many massages, etc. One doctor thought it might be "primary fibromyalgia syndrome" and tried putting me on L-tryptophan and B_6.

All these treatments seemed to help a little at the time, but I still continued to suffer incredible pain.

After my conversation with you, I considered seeing a psychotherapist, but I decided to try it without one first. I came to realize that it was not one big underlying problem causing my tension, but instead any little thing in my daily life that I had learned to fear and/or that caused tension, would begin the cycle of pain, more tension, more pain, etc. If the cause was an unresolved psychological conflict, I noticed that most of the time I didn't actually have to resolve it for the pain to go away but instead just be *aware* that this was the source of my pain. But I do find that now I tend to resolve things more quickly than I did before.

I was so mind-blown and happy over the ability to turn a wrenching spasm into a signal that something must be bothering me (emotionally or mentally) and then dissolve the pain completely within a matter of a minute or less.

It took me four months to get the process under good control, and within less than a year, I was able to say to friends and family, "Yes, my back is finally cured. I am free of pain!"

At the same time that my back became free of pain, so did every single other body part that I mentioned earlier. Finally I could work and play again like I had not done for seven years. What a relief!

I will always be grateful to you, Dr. Sarno, for having the courage and kindness to do what you've been doing for over twenty years—helping people become permanently free of disabling pain.

Thank you.

Dear Dr. John Sarno:

. . . I am greatly improved and now lead a normal active life compared to one of pain and suffering. I do try to inform others whom I think would also benefit from your work.

I just want you to know that you are greatly appreciated by someone who has never met you—but who has been greatly influenced by your special quality.

Again—my heartfelt thanks.

Dear Dr. Sarno:

. . . Reading your book changed my life. I had chronic pain and had tried many "cures," none of which helped until I read your book.

Dear Dr. Sarno:

For six months last year I experienced intense lower back pain. Within two weeks of learning about your TMS theory, my back pain went away. I feel extremely grateful to you and want to tell you my story of your long-distance influence on me.

In July 1988, after jogging one morning, I felt my lower back tighten and a pain radiate down the back of my left leg all the way to my foot. Within twenty-four hours my back hurt so much, I went to my chiropractor. I immediately began following his treatment plan of lying on my back for a few days while icing it as often as possible, followed by beginning mild stretching exercises, stationary bicycling, using a lumbar support, and subsequently a back brace. He told me I had tight muscles, unstable ligaments in the lower spine area, and probably a minor disc injury. I followed this treatment plan faithfully because I trust and like my chiropractor and had experienced successful treatment for previous injuries to my neck and hip muscles. I continued working, lying down frequently and taking short walks regularly.

Unfortunately, the pain did not diminish. Instead it seemed to gradually get worse and worse. For a few weeks in August, while on vacation, I felt mild relief, but when I returned to work, the pain was as bad as ever. I believed, as I was told, that I had injured myself, so I treated myself very carefully: stopped jogging, adjusted my chair at work with lumbar supports, was careful how I moved, and generally began restricting my life since almost everything I did made my back hurt and I was afraid it was interfering with the healing process.

By November, the pain was worse than ever. I began a series of tests in hopes of finding some explanation. My chiropractor did not think anything serious was wrong but was puzzled, along with me, that I was not recovering. I was tested for arthritis, had an X-ray and MRI and a neurological exam. The only result from all this was advice from the neurologist to try swimming—he did not know what was the matter.

By December I was in so much pain that I could barely sit at work and was having trouble concentrating. Since I am a psychotherapist, being able to pay close attention to my clients is essential. With much agony, I decided to take a number of months off work to try to heal myself.

At this point I was desperate for some solution to this problem. Hesitantly, I consulted a psychic. She also told me I had muscle spasms in my back and loose ligaments were preventing them from healing. She recommended acupressure from a Chinese specialist. After five to six sessions of excruciatingly painful treatments, the doctor said (through a translator) that I should be getting better and was puzzled. When he heard I was using ice packs and exercising he said, "Oh, no, you should keep warm, relax and pretend like you're on vacation." Amazingly, after completely relaxing over the weekend, I felt a little relief.

So, the following Monday morning in January (1989)

when I received a letter from an old college friend (who knew about my back) and a copy of an article from *New York* magazine by Tony Schwartz about his miraculous treatment for back pain by a Dr. John Sarno, MD, I was ripe to hear your ideas. I spent the day on the telephone talking to people my friend knew, all who claimed the same miraculous cure . . . and called your office. I was informed I could see you in about six weeks and that you would call in two weeks to set up an appointment.

While I waited I began treating myself. I immediately felt the accuracy of the TMS diagnosis. Consequently it was easy to say to myself that nothing was the matter, I was not injured, the pain was due to tension and it would go away. I also practiced relaxing my back using relaxation meditation techniques and I tried to identify the underlying conflict. Since I have had years of psychotherapy, I was surprised that I would express unconscious conflict somatically. But I decided the conflict had to do with not standing up for myself.

Within two weeks, the pain was gone in relaxed situations. Within two months I was as active as ever. If the pain returned when I went to the movies, I went to the movies every night for a week and told myself the pain would go away. And it did. By the time you called to set up an appointment, I was well on my way to healing and decided I could heal myself.

By May 1989 I discovered the true unconscious conflict causing tension . . . and pain in my back. It became clear that my back pain/tension was part of a group of somatic symptoms occurring during that time (gastrointestinal upset, repeated urinary tract infections, frozen shoulder)

APPENDIX

that were the first signs of my body remembering the tension and pain of early incest experiences.

Over this past year, I have had mild, brief flare-ups of back pain as I resist remembering the painful feelings from sexual abuse. But I know all signs of back pain will be gone when I have healed the psychological wounds.

Let me say again how grateful I am to you. Not only did your ideas provide a framework that allowed me to heal my back pain, but they also contributed to my uncovering the true meaning behind this tension and pain. Now complete healing has begun.

Thank you very much.

INDEX

215

Index

Index

Index

Index

Matthews-Simonton, Stephanie, 186
Mayo Clinic, 146
Migraine headaches, 56, 58, 73, 112, 167–68
  physiology of, 193–95
Millay, Edna St. Vincent, 92
Miller, Neal, 175–76
Mind
  emotional structure of, 163–67
    see also Conscious mind; Emotions; Unconscious mind
  Mind as Healer, Mind as Slayer (Pellatier), 186
Mind-body interactions, 60–68, 155–98
  allergy, 190–91
  and back pain, 6–7, 17–18, 46, 47, 48–50, 57
  and cancer, 186–88
  and cardiovascular system, 175–82
  current research status, 161–63, 174–75
  as defense mechanism, 60–68
  diagnosis, 61
  equivalence principle, 167–69
  and gastrointestinal system, 191–92
  and headache, 193–95
  hypotheses on, 163–73
  and immune system, 182–85
  and infectious diseases, 188–89
  lack of understanding of, 70
  nature of, 164–73
  physicians' problems with, 3, 67, 155–56, 162
  physiochemical concept of pathology, 159–61
  placebo effect, 195–97
  psychologically induced pain, 171–72
  and serious disorders, 172–73
  and skin, 195
  unitary theory of, 171–72
    see also Tension Myositis Syndrome
"Mind Fights Back, The," 188–89
Misinformation, 116

Mitral valve prolapse, 181
Mononeuritis multiplex, 139
Morphine, 145
Motor nerves, 79, 81
MRI. *See* Magnetic resonance imaging
Multiple sclerosis, 184
Muscles
  overworking unused, 111
  oxygen deprivation impact on, 9, 74–76
  relaxation technique, 146–47
  spasm, 16, 18, 22, 76, 208, 212
  strengthening, 149–50
  tenderness in, 7–8
  tension, 204
  TMS involvement, 6–8, 16–17, 117, 126
    see also specific muscles
"Muscle Tissue Oxygen Pressure in Primary Fibromyalgia," 74
Muscular deficiency, 13
Myofascial pain. *See* Fibromyalgia
Myofasciitis. *See* Fibromyalgia
Myofibrositis. *See* Fibromyalgia
Myositis. *See* Tension Myositis Syndrome

Nachemson, Alf, 120
Narcissism, 44–45, 50, 165
National Institutes of Mental Health, 175
Natural History (publication), 196
Neck pain, 6–7, 9, 31, 50, 55, 57, 59, 60, 104–5, 111–12, 116, 139
Nerve blocks, 145
Nerves
  and oxygen deprivation, 10, 78–80
  sciatic, 9, 10, 78–79, 120–54, 170
  spinal, 8–9
  TMS involvement, 8–10, 77–80, 139
    see also Autonomic nervous system; Pinched nerve
Neuritis, 139
Neuroma, 139
Neuroticism, 54, 101, 158–59
New England Journal of Medicine, 68–69, 161
New York magazine, 103, 213

Index

Index

Index

ABOUT THE AUTHOR

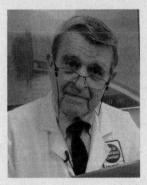

John E. Sarno, MD (1923–2017) was Professor of Rehabilitation Medicine at the New York University School of Medicine. He graduated from Columbia University College of Physicians and Surgeons and was board certified in Physical Medicine and Rehabilitation.

Dr. Sarno served in the U.S. Army Medical Department, 67th Field Hospital-European Theater from 1943 to 1946. He practiced as a family physician for ten years preceding his specialization in rehabilitation medicine. In the early 1950s he initiated the establishment of the Mid-Hudson Medical Group in Fishkill, New York. He served as Director of Outpatient Services and Attending Physician at the Rusk Institute of Rehabilitation Medicine, New York University Medical Center for several decades.